Textbook of
CLINICAL LEPROSY

Textbook of
CLINICAL LEPROSY

FIFTH EDITION

Virendra N Sehgal
MD FNASc FAMS FRAS (Lond)

Consultant/Practicing
Dermato-Venereologist

Visiting Professor
Department of Dermatology and Venereology
Skin Institute and School of Dermatology, Greater Kailash, New Delhi, India

Former
Professor and Head
Department of Dermatology and Venereology
Goa Medical College, Panaji, Goa, India
Professor and Head
Department of Dermatology and Venereology, UCMS
Safdarjung Hospital, New Delhi, India
Professor and Head (Acting Dean), Director-Professor
Department of Dermatology and Venereology
Maulana Azad Medical College/LNJP Hospital, New Delhi, India
Principal and Medical Superintendent/Director-Professor
Department of Dermatology and Venereology
Lady Hardinge Medical College, New Delhi, India
Director-Professor
Department of Dermatology and Venereology
Medical Superintendent, UCMS-GTB Hospital, Delhi, India

JAYPEE BROTHERS MEDICAL PUBLISHERS (P) LTD

New Delhi • Panama City • London • Dhaka • Kathmandu

Jaypee Brothers Medical Publishers (P) Ltd

Headquarters

Jaypee Brothers Medical Publishers (P) Ltd
4838/24, Ansari Road, Daryaganj
New Delhi 110 002, India
Phone: +91-11-43574357
Fax: +91-11-43574314
Email: jaypee@jaypeebrothers.com

Overseas Offices

J.P. Medical Ltd.
83 Victoria Street, London
SW1H 0HW (UK)
Phone: +44-2031708910
Fax: +02-03-0086180
Email: info@jpmedpub.com

Jaypee-Highlights medical publishers Inc.
City of Knowledge, Bld. 237, Clayton
Panama City, Panama
Phone: + 507-301-0496
Fax: + 507-301-0499
Email: cservice@jphmedical.com

Jaypee Brothers Medical Publishers (P) Ltd
17/1-B Babar Road, Block-B, Shaymali
Mohammadpur, Dhaka-1207
Bangladesh
Mobile: +08801912003485
Email: jaypeedhaka@gmail.com

Jaypee Brothers Medical Publishers (P) Ltd
Shorakhute, Kathmandu
Nepal
Phone: +00977-9841528578
Email: jaypee.nepal@gmail.com

Website: www.jaypeebrothers.com
Website: www.jaypeedigital.com

© 2013, Jaypee Brothers Medical Publishers

Inquiries for bulk sales may be solicited at: jaypee@jaypeebrothers.com

This book has been published in good faith that the contents provided by the author contained herein are original, and is intended for educational purposes only. While every effort is made to ensure accuracy of information, the publisher and the author specifically disclaim any damage, liability, or loss incurred, directly or indirectly, from the use or application of any of the contents of this work. If not specifically stated, all figures and tables are courtesy of the author. Where appropriate, the readers should consult with a specialist or contact the manufacturer of the drug or device.

Textbook of Clinical Leprosy

First Edition: 1979
Second Edition: 1987
Third Edition: 1993
Fourth Edition: 2004
Fifth Edition: **2013**

ISBN : 978-93-5090-273-8

Printed at Replika Press Pvt. Ltd.

Dedicated to

*The students, colleagues
and
my wife and grandchildren
Aashna, Vidhvat, Vrishank, Arshia, Rishabh*

Preface to the Fifth Edition

Clinical leprosy, ever since its first publication in the year 1979, has continued to provide an academic access to the understanding of the unique scourge, in tropics including India. Leprosy thus is responsible for making adequate material available for research, despite *Mycobacterium leprae*, its incriminating organism failing to fulfill the Koch's postulates, the major impediment being its denial to grow *in vitro*, thus staking the major breakthrough. Accordingly, the diagnosis of leprosy continues to haunt, and is based primarily on cardinal clinical undertone supplemented by the demonstration of acid-fast-bacilli on slit-skin-smear. Although the latter is a reliable tool, yet it provides only a circumstantial evidence, because it has been repeatedly demonstrated from the lesions of cardinal morphology. Nevertheless, one of the major lacunas is inability to recover the organism on artificial culture. Microscopic pathology seems to surmount this diagnostic dilemma, but it only supplements and not supplant. Hence, it is worthwhile to take cognizance of all the parameters to facilitate its diagnosis, and subsequent treatment in right prospective to curtail the transmission of the disease. The concise facets, therefore, have been imbibed in the text to facilitate clear-cut understanding of the disease. This is an academic exercise, which should meet the requirements of all those interested in the disease.

Virendra N Sehgal

Preface to the First Edition

Leprosy is one of the major public health problems in developing countries. Its teaching should now form an essential content of the undergraduate curriculum in medical institutions in these countries. A clear-cut understanding of clinical manifestations of leprosy is, therefore, imperative. The text of this book deals with different clinical facets of the disease which are essential for the undergraduate and also the postgraduate students. They are based on didactic lectures and clinical demonstration on leprosy, which the author has been imparting to the students for the past two decades. The contents are carefully casted to meet the requirement of curriculum of most institutions. Emphasis has, however, been on the classical clinical features of different types of leprosy. The essentials of diagnosis, and also the treatment have been clearly outlined. The recent concepts of pathogenesis of leprosy, mechanism of reactions, newer drugs and dapsone resistance along with status of leprosy control have been described. The latter, in particular, in Indian subcontinent, has been projected. The generic as well as the trade names of commonly used drugs in leprosy is a unique feature of the text. The book is concise yet comprehensive. It is well-illustrated with neat photographs. It is primarily written to cater to the need of the students, it is hoped, however, that it may be useful also to the practicing physicians, and leprosy field workers, particularly those in developing countries.

Virendra N Sehgal

Acknowledgments

The credit for the success of the first and second editions exclusively rests with the undergraduates and postgraduates, and those practicing with leprosy. I, therefore, express my sincere gratitude to them. The reviewers of the first and third editions of the book are complimented for advancing exquisite suggestions, and pointing out pitfalls and thereby improving and strengthening the text further. They have been imbibed and incorporated in the third edition with pleasure.

It is a pleasure to acknowledge Dr Sanjiv Jain, Practicing Dermatologist, who has assisted me in making invaluable updates throughout the text in order to give a refreshing dimension to match the recent advances on different facets of leprosy. In consequence, the text now gives the book an absolutely new look.

The assistance of Dr Devinder Mohan Thappa and Dr Sambit Nath Bhattacharya, Professor, has been laudable throughout this intriguing task.

Besides, I am grateful to compatriot specialists who have lent helping hands, in propagating and recommending the book to their students.

The art and photographic work was meticulously done by Mr Naresh Kumar and Mr Pravin Kumar and the cover designed by Mr Tilak Raj Gulati of Department of Medical Illustrations, Lady Hardinge Medical College, New Delhi, India. The format of the book was created in the newly established, computerized informatics and research center, Lady Hardinge Medical College.

It was very kind of Dr P Feenstra, Head, Department of Leprosy and TB Control Unit, Royal Tropical Institute, Amsterdam, Netherlands, for permitting the incorporation of 'Basic Requirements for Implementation of Multidrug Therapy'. Besides, the author has taken a liberty to utilize his own published material from various international journals, for which the acknowledgments have been made at appropriate places in the text.

Contents

Historical Background

Leprosy has been known to plague the mankind since times immemorial. Opinions, however, differ over the origin of this disease. Egypt and other middle-east countries enjoy the dubious distinction of having introduced leprosy into the world. Occurrence of leprosy in Egypt dates back to as early as 2400 BC.

India, China and Japan also have been harboring leprosy for thousands of years. *Kustha* cropped up in the writing of Charaka between 600 and 400 BC. Two hundred years later, the term was still retained though with somewhat mutant description. Originally thought to be a specific disease, later on it assumed general form covering a host of different afflictions. Later, the disease was linked with vata-rakta and vata-sonita, characterized by hyperesthesia, anesthesia, formication and other deformities. Furthermore, *kustha* was segregated into *kshudral* (minor) *kustha* and *maha* (major) *kustha*. Similarly, in China, leprosy is known to have occurred as early as 600 BC. However, only in the third century a specific term lai-ping applied to the disease. A definite mention of leprosy is, however, available in Chaon's pathology published around 610 AD. Japanese records date back to 400 BC and indicate disseminated existence of leprosy in historic times.

Leprosy was introduced into the Mediterranean countries around 467 BC and 150 AD between the era of Hippocrates and Galen; by that time the disease was well-known. Leprosy, then, appears to have propogated unabated because of lack of any knowledge of its control and treatment. Subsequently, it acquired considerable heights in Europe between 1000 and 1400 AD. To the American continent, leprosy is thought to be carried through Columbus and his soldiers and also by the slave trade from highly endemic areas in West Africa.

1

Mycobacterium Leprae

The causative organism of leprosy is *Mycobacterium leprae*. It was isolated as intracellular microorganism in the smears from leprosy nodules in 1874. It is an acid-fast bacillus. Morphologically, it is a straight or slightly curved, slender bacillus, about the size of 5×0.5 mμ with pointed, rounded or club shaped ends. It is non-sporing and is less strongly acid-fast than *Mycobacterium tuberculosis*. It resists decolorization with five percent sulphuric acid (Figs 1.1 to 1.3). The bacilli usually stain evenly, but irregular staining is also seen in smears from patients on dapsone. The latter is characterized by beadings. The proportion of evenly staining to irregularly staining bacilli is an important laboratory test, and is known as *morphological index*. It helps in the assessment of the effectiveness of chemotherapy in leprosy. The organism is gram-positive, and can be stained instantly by Grams' stain.

The organism has not yet been grown on any artificial culture media. It has, however, been inoculated in the footpad of thymectomized and irradiated mice. The bacilli in due course invade the nerves, skin and other tissues of mice. Hence, this has been utilized for assessing the chemotherapy of leprosy at some centers.

The bacilli are present in the skin, nerves and other tissues in lepromatous, borderline (dimorphous) and also tuberculoid leprosy. But their demonstration is easy in slit-skin smears in lepromatous and borderline leprosy. The procedure for the slit-skin smear is very simple, and is

described here. The preparation of smear and its staining should form an office procedure.

Slit-skin smear: The smears are prepared from scrapings from a skin infection of the lesion, particularly of the ear lobe, which may yield a

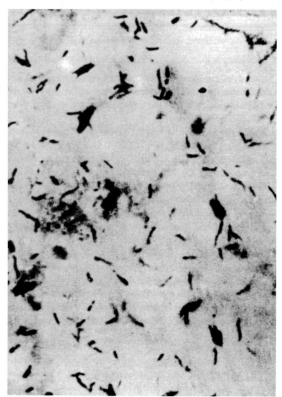

Fig 1.1: *Mycobacterium leprae* (oil immersion × 1000)

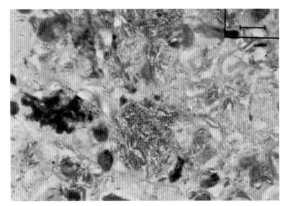

Fig 1.2: Numerous scattered as well as grouped acid-fast bacilli (Ziehl-Neelsen stain x 1000)

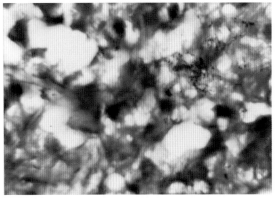

Fig 1.3: Tissue sections displaying histocytes-globi-containing acid fast lepra bacilli (Ziehl-Neelson stain x 1000)

positive result even when there is no obvious local lesion. The smears are also made from any ulcerated nodule on the skin or a non-ulcerated nodule may be punctured with the needle and squeezed until serum exudes.

The slit-skin smears are stained by Ziehl-Neelsen stain according to the following procedure.

Ziehl-Neelsen stain: The slit-skin smears are dried and fixed by passing over a flame. The slide is covered with filtered carbolfuchsin and heated until steam rises. The preparation is allowed to stain for five minutes, heat being applied at intervals to keep the stain hot, also taking care that the stain does not dry up.

The slide is then washed under running water followed by decolorization with five percent sulfuric acid. The red color of the preparation changes to yellowish brown. Repeated pouring of the acid, with alternate washing may be required for complete decolorization of the preparation, which is indicated by faint pink color of the film. This procedure may require ten minutes to complete.

The slide at this stage is washed again in running water. It is followed by treating the slide with 96 percent alcohol for a period of two minutes, followed by immediate washing again with water. Now the preparation is ready for counter staining which is done with methylene blue for a period of 15 to 20 seconds.

The preparation is blotted, dried and mounted for the demonstration of lepra bacilli. They are recognized by their morphological characteristics as described above. The grading of smears is done as outlined below:

One to 10 bacilli in 100 fields	(1+)
One to 10 bacilli in 10 fields	(2+)
One to 10 bacilli in average fields	(3+)
Ten to 100 bacilli in average fields	(4+)
Hundred to 1000 bacilli in average field	(5+)
Clumps and globi in average field	(6+)

Bacterial Index (BI): It is calculated by totalling the number of plus (+) given to each smear and dividing the same by the number of smears collected. The accuracy of this examination results from examination a minimum of four skin lesions, nasal swabs and both the ear lobes, namely,

Right ear	++
Left ear	+++
Nasal smear	++
First skin lesion	++
Second skin lesion	++
Third skin lesion	++
Fourth skin lesion	+
Total number of sites examined	= 7
Total number of plus (+)	= 14
Bacterial Index	= 14/7 = 2

Morphological Index (MI): It is an useful procedure to evaluate the effectiveness of antileprosy therapy. This is determined by counting the number of both the regularly and irregularly stained bacilli in the smear. Only bacilli showing uniform staining throughout their length should be considered regularly stained. The count should preferably be done on a total of 100 or more organisms in fields picked at random. *Morphological Index (MI)* is calculated as number of regularly stained bacilli per hundred of total organisms examined, for example:

Total number of organisms examined	= 100
Number of regularly stained bacilli	= 10
Morphological index	= 10 percent

Fluorescence microscopy: This may also be used for demonstration of lepra bacilli. It is based on alcohol acid-fastness of bacilli where the fuchsin which is used in Ziehl-Neelsen method is replaced by auramine or its derivatives. Ultraviolet light is used for fluorescence. The bacilli appear yellow and bright on the dark background and are easily detected with lower magnification. Furthermore, the field observed is very large and the smear can be examined rapidly. This method is especially useful for laboratories with very heavy workload of smear examination.

LEPROMIN TEST

It is performed by intracutaneous injection of 0.1 ml of 'standard' lepromin—an antigen produced from lepromatous granuloma. It should contain 160 million lepra bacilli per ml. It is prepared by using 4–5 g of lepromatous tissue to get a final suspension of 100 ml. It should be free from visible tissue particles, and could be diluted for use. One in four dilutions containing 40 million bacilli per ml, is adequate to produce nodule of 3 mm or more in four weeks, a criterion for its positivity.

The reaction may either be early (Fernandez) or delayed (mitsuda).

Early (Fernandez) reaction: It develops in 24 to 48 hours and lasts three to five days. The formation of erythema and induration characterize the reaction. Following are the criteria for its reading:

Induration less than 5 mm	
Induration more than 5 mm	±
Induration more than 10 mm	+
Induration more than 15 mm	+ +
Induration more than 20 mm	+ + +

Delayed (Mitsuda) reaction: In leprosy patients and contacts, it should be recorded at four weeks. In others, it should be recorded and read in four to five weeks. In any case, if the reaction is negative or doubtful, further reading should be recorded at seven to nine weeks. The criteria for reading the results are as follows:

No reaction	0
Induration less than 3 mm	+
Nodule of 3 mm to 5 mm	+
Nodule of 6 mm to 10 mm	+ +
Nodule of larger than 10 mm or with ulceration	+ + +

The letter 'U' should be added to the size to indicate ulceration.

SIGNIFICANCE OF LEPROMIN TEST

The significance of this test lies only in assessing the immunological status of an individual suffering from leprosy, and in contacts. It is one plus (+) to three plus (+ + +) positive in maculo anesthetic and tuberculoid, while is negative (–) to (+) in lepromatous and borderline leprosy respectively. The Mitsuda reaction is due to cell-mediated immunity.

RECOMMENDED READING

1. Dharmendra. Bacteriological examination. In: Notes on leprosy. Delhi: Ministry of Health, Govt. of India. 1967;311-316.
2. Leiker DL, McDougall AC. Technical guide for smear examination for leprosy, *Leprosy Documentation Services*, Amsterdam, 1983;7:29.
3. Ridely DS. Bacterial indices. In: Cochrane RG, (Ed). Leprosy in theory and practice, Bristol; John Wright and Sons, 1959;371.
4. Ridley DS. The SFG (Solid, fragmental, granular) index for bacterial morphology. *Lepr Rev.* 1971; 42:96-97.
5. Sehgal VN, Joginder. Slit-skin smear in leprosy. *Int J Dermatol.* 1990;29:9-16.
6. Wade HW. Examination of skin smears for bacilli (editorial). *Int J Lepr.* 1965;31:240-242.
7. Waters MF, Rees RJ. Changes in the morphology of *Mycobacterium leprae* in patients under treatment. *Int J Lepr.* 1962;30:266-277.

2

Epidemiology of Leprosy

Epidemiology of leprosy is an intriguing subject, for many of its parameters till date present some features, parallel of which are not found in other diseases. Nevertheless, a satisfactory explanation is not forthcoming because of inability to culture the causative organism *Mycobacterium leprae* and to study its behavior. It is, however, imperative to understand the factors responsible for perpetuating the disease, in relation to both the causative organisms and the host.

GLOBAL DISTRIBUTION

Leprosy is a chronic infective disease found throughout the world, and its total estimate is not precisely known. However, it is believed that more than 10,786,000 people are suffering from this scourge. Its prevalence is fairly alarming in India and China and is highest in Africa. In India alone, there are more than 3.2 million people suffering from this disease. Figure 2.1 depicts the worldwide distribution and prevalence of leprosy.

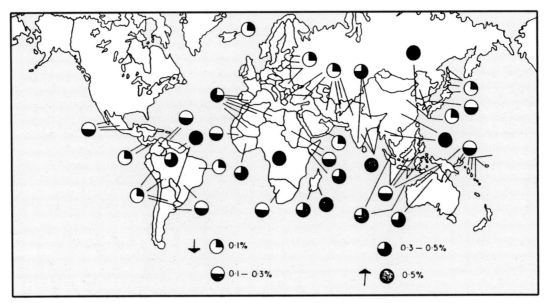

Fig. 2.1: Global distribution of leprosy

DISTRIBUTION IN INDIA

The leprosy patients are generally seen all over India in endemic form; however, stray cases are seen in Punjab, Chandigarh, Delhi and Andaman and Nicobar Islands. It is prevalent in the southern and eastern states. The states of high endemicity with over 1 per cent leprosy are—Tamil Nadu, Andhra Pradesh, West Bengal, Orissa, Bihar, Maharashtra, Karnataka, Pondicherry, Eastern Utter Pradesh and Assam. The moderately endemic states are Madhya Pradesh, Gujrat, Kerala, Himachal Pradesh, Meghalaya, Manipur, Nagaland, Mizoram, Tripura, Goa, Daman and Diu, and Dadra and Nagar Haveli, where the incidence of leprosy varies from 0.5 percent to below 1 percent. The states like Jammu and Kashmir, Haryana, Rajasthan and Lakshadweep island are low endemic states, where the incidence of leprosy is 0.1 to 0.5 percent. However, there are some hyperendemic areas and foci in the moderate and low endemic states also as detailed in Figure 2.2.

CHANGING SCENARIO

The current strategy for eliminating leprosy revolves around, and is based on the presumption that once the prevalence of less than 1/10,000 is achieved through the institution of multidrug therapy (MDT) at the global level, it is likely to diminish the transmission, and may eventually wipe out the

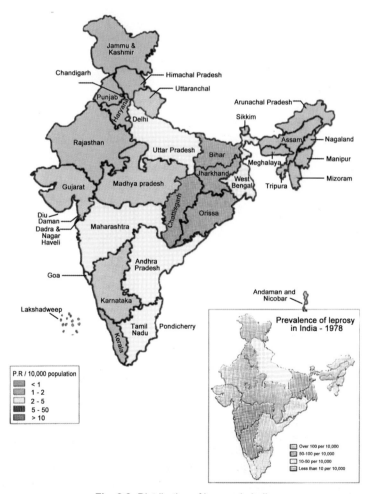

Fig. 2.2: Distribution of leprosy in India

disease. This assumption is derived from the fact that MDT is capable of accomplishing this objective is yet to be complied with. Using registered prevalence as a proxy indicator for the epidemiology of leprosy has several caveats. By definition it only reflects registered cases, and thus obscures true leprosy cases reported to private practitioners or practicing specialists. The prevalence taken for leprosy control is point prevalence and not a period prevalence. The incidence of the disease is therefore better monitor, but so far no data are available on incidence rates. However, case detection rates (CDR) are available for leprosy, but are far from good indicators of incidence. The CDR is likely to be inflated by backlog cases, and/or defaulting and relapse cases. Moreover; it is heavily influenced by intensity of case finding effects. Trends in CDR may thus be distorted as a result of bias and confounding. CDR trends at a global level may be relatively stable, while at a country level CDRs may show a declining, stable or even a rising trend.

The fact that *M. leprae* cannot be cultured *in vitro*; it is impossible to assess the exposure, and the onset of the disease. The chain of infection, considered as the relationship between *M. leprae* transmission, and the human host, is poorly understood as of today (Fig. 2.3).

Reservoir of Infection

An infectious-open case, comprising lepromatous, borderline leprosy is mainly the reservoir of infection, but the so-called closed cases of leprosy consisting of tuberculoid and other types may also act as a source.

Transmission

Leprosy is transmitted from person to person by close contact with an infected individual. However, sometimes a short contact may also cause transmission of the disease. Occasionally, infected syringes, tattooing needles, vaccinations and fomites also transmit this disease.

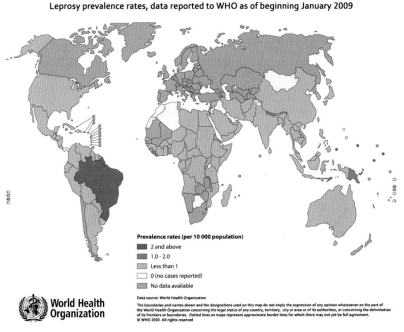

Fig. 2.3: Global and regional map showing prevalence of Leprosy at the start of 2010
(*Courtesy:* World Health Organization)

Portal of Entry

The organism usually enters the body of the host through an apparently normal or abraded skin. The mucous membrane of the upper respiratory tract may also be amenable. Further, the gastrointestinal tract may also serve as portal of entry.

Incubation Period

It is hard to define the incubation period of leprosy for it is difficult to elicit a history of contact with an infected individual. All the same, it is thought to vary from a few months to many years.

▮ AGE AT ONSET

In leprosy, it is not possible to determine the age at infection until a reliable test is developed. Hence, the age at onset is used as an approximate guide to find the susceptible groups. The approximate age at onset is worked out by subtracting the duration of the disease from the reporting age. The duration of the disease is determined by inquiring from the patient, family members and associates, about the earliest, clinical manifestations of the disease. The age at onset is variable. It differs from country to country and region to region in the same country due to various known and unknown factors. Furthermore, the age at onset varies according to type of leprosy, being lowest is tuberculoid and highest in polyneuritic, while in borderline and lepromatous cases, it is in between (Fig. 2.4).

The common reporting age in children is between 5 and 14 years and in adults 20 and 59 years.

▮ SEX PREVALENCE

Both males and females contract leprosy; preponderance of the former is the common observation. However, the sex prevalence is one of the various factors, namely immigration, opportunity for contact and social customs. In endemic belts of the world and in developing countries, the chances of contact with infected person(s) are more or less

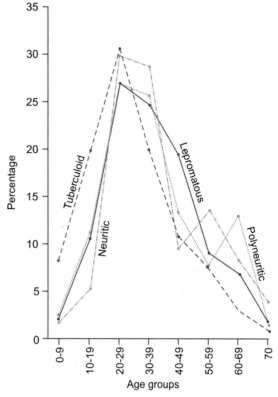

Fig. 2.4: Age of onset of leprosy

equal. Hence, in these countries, no difference may be observed in males and females. It may also be influenced by stringent social customs and taboos. Urbanization and industrialization may also influence the sex prevalence directly or due to immigration. The latter may also hold good for affluent and developed countries.

▮ FAMILY INCIDENCE

It depends on several factors, namely, the occurrence of the disease in the family and opportunities of close contact with the family members. It is believed that larger the numbers of individuals in a family residing in a meager accommodation, greater are the chances for contracting the disease. Family incidence may in turn determine the prevalence of the disease in the community.

▌ INDIVIDUAL FACTORS

The susceptibility of the individuals to *Mycobacterium leprae* may show variations and are determined by the immunological response. An individual may be capable of resisting the invading organism without showing any clinical or histopathological manifestations or it may allow the organism to gain a foot-hold in the body in either a limited or a generalized way. The individual capable of producing the cell-mediated immunity (CMI) localize or focalize the disease-tuberculoid leprosy, while in those where CMI is lacking, the disease becomes generalized-lepromatous leprosy.

The immunological phenomenon may be responsible for the different patterns of the disease seen around the world. In India and Africa, tuberculoid leprosy forms the bulk of the cases, but in Burma and China, the majority of cases are lepromatous. Likewise, higher incidence of polyneuritic leprosy and nerve abscesses are peculiar to India.

Climate

Leprosy is known to be prevalent in tropical and subtropical regions of the world, but there is no conclusive evidence to support the role of climate in the epidemiology of leprosy. It is likely that other factors, e.g. general health, diet, socioeconomic status, customs and housing in these regions, may be contributory to its prevalence.

Race

It seems that race has also been incriminated in the prevalence of leprosy though without any favorable evidence. It may be attributed to a variety of factors like opportunity of contact and susceptibility. In this connection, it is worthwhile to mention that certain races like Mongolian and European are more prone to develop lepromatous leprosy than African and Indian.

Diet

There is no adequate evidence that leprosy is in any way due to dietetic deficiencies or does it appears to play any major part in its epidemiology.

▌ RECOMMENDED READING

1. Anonymous. Epidemiology of leprosy in relation to control. Technical Report Series no. 716, Geneva, World Health Organisation, 1985;21.
2. Fine PE. Reflections on the elimination of leprosy. *Int J Lepr Other Mycobact Dis*. 1992;60:71-80.
3. Leprosy. Fact sheet no. 101. Geneva, World Health Organization, January 2001.
4. Sehgal VN, Joginder. Tuberculoid (TT) leprosy; localization on a tattoo. *Lepr Rev*. 1989;60:241-242.
5. Sehgal VN. Inoculation leprosy. Current status. *Int J Dermatol*, 1988;27:6-9.
6. Visschedik J, Van de Broek J, Eggens H, Lever P, Van Beers S, Klatser P. Mycobacterium leprae-millennium resistant. Leprosy control on the threshold of a new era. *Tropical Med Int Health*. 2000;5:388–399.

CHAPTER 3

Pathogenesis, Pathology and Evolution of Classification

Until the discovery of *Mycobacterium leprae* in 1874, the pathogenesis of clinical manifestations of leprosy was hardly understood. The discovery gave an impetus to workers in different disciplines of medicine to probe into its intricacies. The concept which has evolved today as a result is debatable yet comprehensive, because largely it provides a well framed correlation between the clinical, histopathological and immunological aspects of the disease.

Mycobacterium leprae is the causative organism of the disease. It is transmitted from person-to-person by direct, prolonged and intimate skin-to-skin contact, usually with an open (infectious) case of leprosy. Occasionally, indirect contact through infected syringe, tattooing needles, and fomites has also been known to transmit the disease. The usual portal of entry is an apparently normal or abraded skin/mucous membrane. The respiratory and the gastrointestinal tract may also act as a portal of entry. Arthropods are again being incriminated in the transmission of the disease. The organism may encounter a favorable or unfavorable environment in the host.

The unfavorable environment may succeed in extricating the organisms from the body without any manifest clinical features. The sequences of events are outlined in Figure 3.1. Nevertheless, the presence of the organisms may be demonstrated in the proliferating monocytes. This forms the silent

phase seen in the contacts, and they may be lepromin positive.

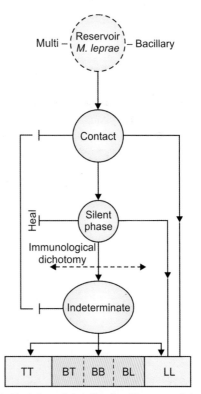

Fig. 3.1: Evolution of classification (*Courtesy:* Sehgal VN and Srivastava G. *Lepr. Rev*, 1997;58:291)

INDETERMINATE LEPROSY

In the favorable environment, on the other hand, the organisms may gain a foot-hold and gradually start multiplying and spread toward the nerve endings for which they have an affirmity. At this stage, the body defenses compromising lymphocytes and histiocytes are mobilized around the nerve fibers. Clinically, if may manifest in the form of an early ill defined macule(s) of indeterminate leprosy.

Histopathology of these lesions may reveal lymphocytic and histiocytic infiltrate around the adnexa, and the blood vessels (Fig. 3.2) perineural infiltration, however, is a significant diagnostic feature.

The course of indeterminate leprosy is variable. It may remain quiescent, recover spontaneously or progress insidiously. Its further progress depends upon the immunological responses of the body. It may then lead to lepromatous, tuberculoid or an unstable group of leprosy.

LEPROMATOUS LEPROSY

In individual where the resistance is low-evident clinically as lepromin negative—the lepra bacilli take the upper hand, and cross the cordon of inflammatory infiltrate to reach the terminal nerve endings. They are taken up by the regenerating nerves for which they have an affinity. They

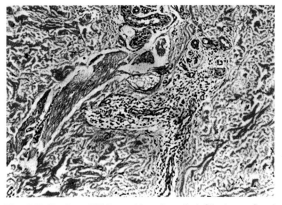

Fig. 3.2: Scattered histo-and lymphocytic infiltrate confined to appendages and blood vassels, suggesting indeterminate leprosy (H & E x 250)

rapidly multiply in the columns of Schwann cells, enveloping the individual nerve fiber. In the process, they produce sacculations in the nerve sheath.

The sacculations may burst and disseminate the organisms into the surrounding tissue spaces. At this stage, the organisms enter the blood stream so that the disease becomes generalized. In the tissues, the organisms are engulfed by the histiocytes. The organisms continue to proliferate in these cells, giving rise to small to large vacuoles forming the so-called Virchows' or foam cells. Furthermore, these cells may enlarge and burst, scattering the bacilli to be taken up by other histiocytes.

The brunt of the infection is borne by the nerves, skin, mucous membranes, reticuloendothelial system, and tests.

In the early stages of the disease, there is hardly any structural damage to the nerve; this may last for a number of years, coinciding probably with the incubation period of leprosy. Later, edema, fibrosis and hyaline degeneration may develop in the peripheral nerves, significantly without any inflammatory cellular infiltrate. The large nerve trunks may also undergo thickening and form fusiform, beaded or diffuse swellings.

Skin histology is characterized by the scattered granuloma comprising foam cells interspersed with a few lymphocytes. The foamy change is variable from small to large vacuoles. The presence of clear, subepidermal zone is characteristic. The nerves may be unaffected or show the onion-peel perineurium without much infiltration. The acid-fast lepra bacilli are abundant, arranged singly, in clumps or globi (Figs 3.3 and 3.4).

Similar changes are noted in the mucous membranes. The circulating organisms, in the process are also trapped by the reticuloendothelial system comprising the lymph nodes, liver, spleen, and bone marrow. The granulomas in these organs resemble those of the skin. The testes are affected as orchitis and the granulomas are present in the interstitial tissues under the capsule, mediastinum testis and setae between the lobules. This may gradually be replaced by fibrous tissues leading to atrophy and hardening of the glands.

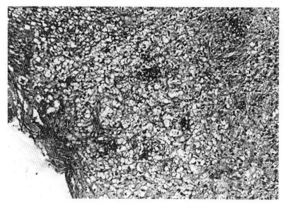

Fig. 3.3: Scattered granulomas formed by foamy macrophages and scanty lympocytes displaying lepromatous lepromatous leprosy (H & E x 160)

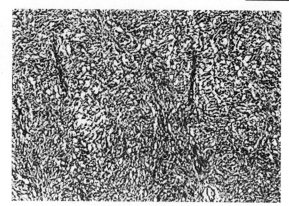

Fig. 3.4: Another section decpicting the lepromatous lepromatous features (H & E x 10)

Criteria for diagnosis of Lepromatous Lepromatous (LL)

I. The formation of scattered granuloma containing numerous foamy macrophages in the lower dermis
II. The clear zone is well-marked.
III. The nerves are preserved and have as 'onion-peel' appearance.
IV. The acid-fast bacilli are numerous and are found throughout the granuloma.
V. AFB 5–6.

Histoid Leprosy

It is a variant of multibacillary leprosy, also designated as 'mixed lepromatous'. Its aetiopathogenesis is not precisely known. Histology is, however, quite characteristic. The granuloma is formed of spindle-shaped histiocytes containing acid-fast bacilli with little or no cell vacuolization (Figs 3.5 and 3.6).

Tuberculoid Leprosy

The indeterminate or silent phase of leprosy may progress to form tuberculoid leprosy, where the host resistance is high as depicted by a strongly positive lepromin test. The lepra bacilli enter the Schwann cells, which soon become fixed epitheliod cells due to high immune response. These cells are capable of killing and lysing the bacilli. In due course, a group of epitheliod cells appears inside the fine nerve twigs surrounded by lymphocytes, and histiocytes. Some of the epitheloid cells unite to form langhan's type of giant cells. The intraneural infiltration may lead to destruction of the structure of the nerve twigs. The disease may remain only intraneural—pure neural tuberculoid leprosy— wherein the affected nerve(s) become thickened and painful. The motor and sensory modalities may get involved consequently. At times caseation necrosis in the nerves may form localized swellings-nerve abscess (Figs 3.7 and 3.8).

The bacilli may invade the skin to form a lesion at the site. The microscopic pathology of the skin lesions is characterized by epitheliod cell granulomas, surrounded by densely packed lymphocytes. The granulomas usually invade and destroy the epidermis-epidermal erosions. The presence of Langhan's giant cell, central caseation and massive enlargement of nerve bundles surrounded by a zone of lymphocytes and absence of a subepidermal zone are its salient feature. Acid-fast lepra bacilli are difficult to demonstrate.

The regional cutaneous nerve supplying the skin lesions of tuberculoid leprosy may be thickened and tender.

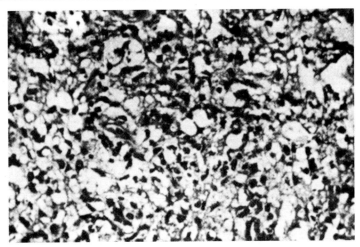

Fig. 3.5: Histoid leprosy: Spindle-shaped histiocytes containing acid-fast bacilli with little or no cell vacuolization (H & E x 100)

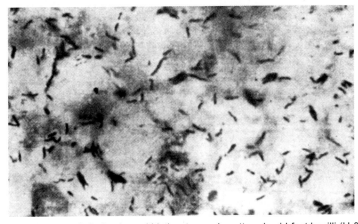

Fig. 3.6: Histoid leprosy: Spindle-shaped histiocytes and scattered acid-fast bacilli (H & E x 100)

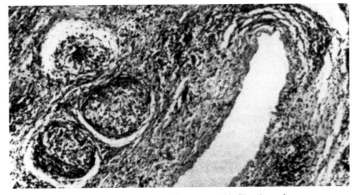

Fig. 3.7: Polyneuritic leprosy: Intraneural infiltration of nerves
(*Courtesy:* Sehgal VN, *et al. Int J Lep,* 1967;35:60)

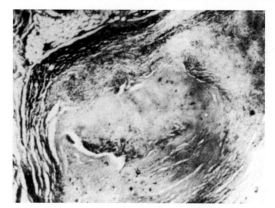

Fig. 3.8: Nerve abscess: caseation necrosis (H & E x 100)

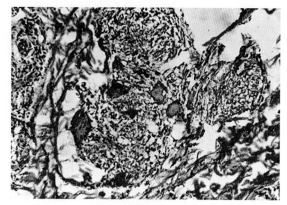

Fig. 3.9

> **Criteria for histopathological classification of Tuberculoid Tuberculoid (TT) (Figs 3.9 to 3.11)**
>
> I. Compact granuloma of epitheliod cells, giant cells, and a large number of lymphocytes.
> II. The granuloma is located just beneath the epidermis extending to mid-dermis.
> III. In addition, the infiltrate is also present in the epidermis-epidermal erosion.
> IV. Infiltration and complete destruction of cutaneous nerves is a constant feature (Nerve are unidentifiable).
> V. The acid-fast *Mycobacterium leprae* is, however, difficult to demonstrate.
> VI. AFB 0–1.

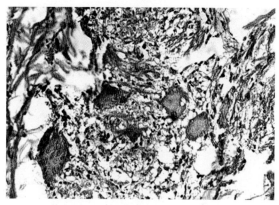

Fig. 3.10

Figs 3.9 and 3.10: Compact granuloma containing epitheloid cells, large number of lymphocytes and giant cells, occupying the upper dermis, displaying the microscopic pathology of tuberculoid tuberculoid leprosy (H & E x 160 and 250)

▌ BORDERLINE LEPROSY

The transformation of indeterminate to borderline leprosy seems to be a frequent occurrence. It happens in the subject with unstable host resistance. The morphological characteristics of this group are, therefore, variable and may show features of both tuberculoid and lepromatous leprosy with predominance of one or the other. The lepromin test may also show variations—from negative to weakly positive. It may evolve into one or the other polar types.

Epithelioid cell granulomas, scanty lymphocytes and a clear subepidermal zone are the main histological presentations (Fig. 3.12). The nerves

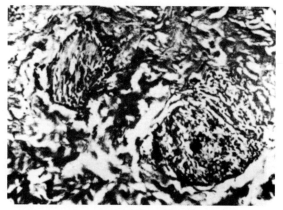

Fig. 3.11: Tuberculoid leprosy: Massive infiltration of the nerves (H & E x 100)

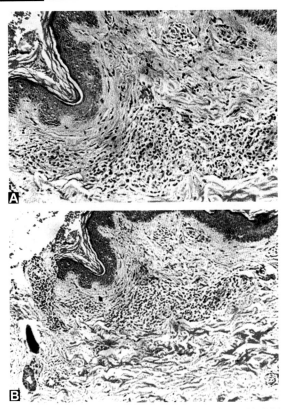

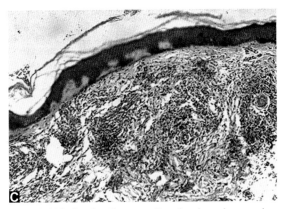

Figs 3.12A and B: Diffuse granuloma comprising epitheloid cells, scanty lymphocytes, no giant cells and a free subepidermal zone, suggesting borderline leprosy (H & E x 160 and 250)

Fig. 3.12C: Another tissue section showing microscopic features of borderline leprosy (H & E x 160)

may be normal or may be swollen by the cellular infiltrate; acid-fast bacilli can easily be detected. A shift toward the tuberculoid pole is suggested by the formation of a foreign body or Langhans' type of giant cells, a tendency to obliterate the clear zone and reduction in the number of lepra bacilli (Figs 3.13 and 3.14). A shift toward the lepromatous pole, on the other hand, is indicated by the appearance of macrophages (Figs 3.15 and 3.16). The lymphocytes may be arranged in dense clumps. There is an increase in the number of acid-fast bacilli, which may also be demonstrable in the infiltrated cutaneous nerves.

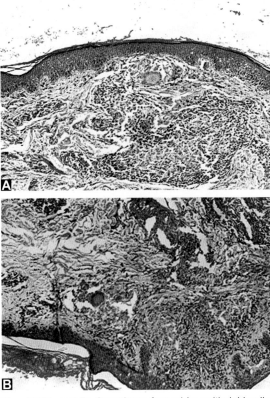

Figs 3.13A and B: Granuloma formed by epitheloid cells, plenty of lymphocytes and a giant cell, narrow, relatively free, subepidermal zone conforming to borderline tuberculoid histology (H & E x 160 and 400)

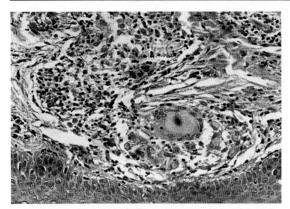

Fig. 3.14: Another tissue section depicting borderline tuberculoid (H & E x 160)

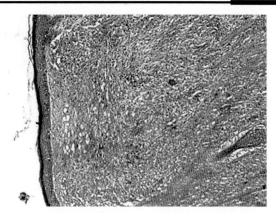

Fig. 3.15: Diffuse granuloma of histocytes, formation of macrophages-foam cells-with clumps of lymphocytes suggesting borderline lepromatous leprosy (H & E x 160)

Criteria for histological diagnosis of borderline leprosy Borderline Tuberculoid (BT)

I. Granuloma formed by epitheliod cells and plentiful of lymphocytes. Giant cells are either absent or occasional.

II. Dermal nerves are swollen with infiltrate, but are recognizable.

III. AFB 0–2.

Borderline Borderline (BB)

I. The appearance of granuloma is marked by the presence of epitheliod cells, absence of giant cells and scanty lymphocytes scattered all over the granuloma.

II. The formation of a relatively free subepidermal zone.

III. The texture of the nerves is generally maintained through they had infiltration of epitheliod cells.

IV. The acid-fast lepra bacilli are easily demonstrable.

V. AFB 3–4.

Borderline Lepromatous (BL)

I. The presence of granuloma comprising histiocytes, sheets of lymphocytes and macrophages containing acid-fast bacilli. The granuloma is diffuse and located in the mid-and lower dermis.

II. The presence of eosinophilic staining zone below the epidermis is conspicuous.

III. The structure of the nerves is maintained and is infiltrated by histiocytes. The classical "onion-peel" is the landmark in the diagnosis.

IV. The acid-fast lepra bacilli are easily identifiable in the sections stained with Ziehl-Neelsen's method.

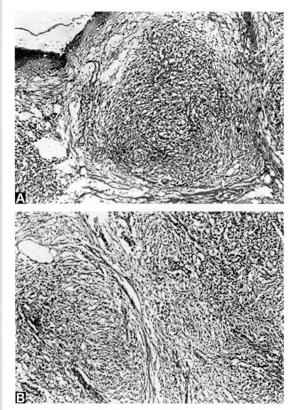

Figs 3.16A and B: Tissue sections showing the identical features (H & E x 160)

▮ RECOMMENDED READING

1. Sehgal VN, Koranne RV, Nayyar M, Saxena HM. Application of clinical and histopathological

classification of leprosy. *Dermatologica.* 1980;161:93-96.

2. Sehgal VN, Koranne RV, Sehgal S, Beoher PC, Sharma VK. Correlation of morphological, bacteriological, histopathological and immunological features of leprosy. A double blind study. *J Dermatol.* 1985;12:243-250.

3. Sehgal VN, Rege VL, Reys M. Correlation between clinical, and histopathologic classification of leprosy. *Int J Lepr Other Mycobact Dis.* 1977;45:278-280.

4. Sehgal VN, Srivastava G, Singh N, Prasad PV. Histoid leprosy; the impact of the entity on post-global leprosy elimination era. *Int J Dermatol.* 2009;48:603-610.

5. Sehgal VN, Srivastava G, Singh N. Histoid leprosy: histopathological connotations relevance in contemporary context. *Am J Dermatopathol.* 2009;31:268-271.

6. Sehgal VN, Srivastava G. Indeterminate leprosy. A passing phase in the evolution of leprosy. *Lepr Rev.* 1987;58:291-299.

Immunology of Leprosy

It is indeed intriguing that a spectrum of clinical disease is produced by identical strains of *Mycobacterium leprae*, reflecting that immune status of the host largely determine whether after infection percent the patient would be successful in eradicating the bacteria or develop indeterminate (I) leprosy which may remain as such, resolve, or progress to the determinate forms. These may be tuberculoid tuberculoid (TT), borderline tuberculoid (BT), borderline borderline (BB), borderline lepromatous (BL) and lepromatous leprosy (LL). Hence, it is imperative to comprehend the immune responses in leprosy. The immune response is responsible for the defense against infections. The outcome of the interaction between the infecting microorganism and the immunity reflects host resistance. The immunity is either humoral or cellular, mediated by immunoglobulins and T lymphocytes respectively. Although both forms of immune responses are activated in leprosy, it is the cellular immunity which is significant, as *M. leprae*, is intracellular. If the host mounts an adequate cell-mediated immunity (CMI) against the organism, the disease is restricted to the tuberculoid end. In its absence, the infection becomes generalized and the patient moves toward the lepromatous end.

The nature of CMI deficiency in leprosy is a matter of speculation. It may either be specific CMI deficiency towards *M. leprae*, or combined specific and nonspecific impairment of CMI. The nonspecific immunity may be restored after initiating therapy.

LEPROMIN TEST

This reflects the CMI responses of the individual to *M. leprae*. It is strongly positive in tuberculoid and negative in lepromatous leprosy. It is weakly positive or negative in borderline group. Various antigens used in lepromin test are:

1. Integral lepromin consisting of crude suspension of leprous tissue.
2. Dharmendra antigen consisting of defatted bacillary suspension.
3. Leprolin consisting of soluble protein of bacilli.

The antigens may be prepared from the lesions of armadillo (lepromin A) or form human tissue (lepromin H). The response to lepromin H containing 100 million bacilli per ml is equivalent to 1 ml of lepromin. A having 40 million bacilli.

Lepromin test may either be read at 24 to 48 hours (Fernandez reaction) and at 4 weeks (Mitsuda reaction). Fernandez reaction is attributed to cross reaction with other mycobacteriae whereas, Mitsuda reaction provides a better reflection of CMI to *M. leprae*.

EPICUTANEOUS SENSITIZATION TO DINITROCHLOROBENZENE (DNCB)

The ability to develop contact sensitivity to DNCB is a good indicator of T-cell immunity and also helps to differentiate whether impairment is minimal in tuberculoid and maximum in lepromatous leprosy. The response may improve during reversal reactions.

T Lymphocytes and its Subsets in Peripheral Blood

A step ladder decrease in total T cell count and percentage has been found from tuberculoid to lepromatous end of the spectrum. T-lymphocytes may be depleted from paracortical areas of lymph nodes in lepromatous leprosy. T4/T8 ratio has been observed to be normal in tuberculoid leprosy and either decrease or unaltered in lepromatous leprosy.

T Lymphocytes and Subsets in Leprosy Lesion

T-helper cells predominate in tuberculoid granuloma while in the lepromatous granuloma T-suppressor cells out number T-helper cells. In tuberculoid granuloma, the T-suppressor cells from a lymphocytic mantle around the granuloma whereas T-helper cells are diffusely scattered. No such segregation of T-cell subpopulation has been observed in tuberculoid granuloma whereas they are scanty in lepromatous leprosy.

Macrophages

Macrophages are unable to destroy *M. leprae* in lepromatous leprosy, while in tuberculoid patients this function is intact. A failure of antigen presentation by macrophages to T-lymphocytes is a feature in lepromatous leprosy.

Interleukins

Macrophages on coming contact with foreign antigen liberate interleukin-I. This activates the antigens specific T-cells. Interleukin-I induces a set of specific T-cells to produce T-cell growth factor, interleukin-2, along with interleukin-2 receptors (IL-2R) on other T-lymphocytes. The interaction between soluble interleukin-2 and its receptors results in proliferation of T-lymphocytes to combat the antigen. The unresponsiveness of lepromatous leprosy to *M. leprae* is attributed to failure to produce IL-2. This results in failure of T-cell clonal proliferation and subsequent destruction and removal of the bacteria.

B-Lymphocytes in Peripheral Blood

B cell count is normal in tuberculoid, high in lepromatous leprosy and intermediate in borderline group.

Serum Immunoglobulins

As in other chronic infective disorder, a raised level of gamma globulins is observed in leprosy. The levels are significantly higher in lepromatous as compared to tuberculoid leprosy.

Immunological Dichotomy

The dual immunological responses in leprosy are aptly described as immunologic dichotomy. Its characteristic features are outlined in Table 4.1.

Table 4.1: Characteristic of immunological dichotomy	
1. Adequate cell-mediated immunity	1. Impaired cell-mediated immunity
2. Limited bacillary multiplication	2. Myriads of bacilli
3. Localized, well-defined, circumscribed lesions	3. Extensive diffuse, poorly delimited lesions
4. Delayed hypersensitivity to intradermal testing with nonspecific antigens such as candida, tuberculin, mumps and histoplasmin	4. Energy to intradermal testing with the nonspecific antigens
5. Sensitization to dinitrochlorobenzene (DNCB)	5. Impaired or absent response to DNCB
6. Strongly positive lymphocytes transformation test (LTT) to *M. leprae* antigen	6. Negative LTT

Contd...

Contd...

7. Strongly positive lymphocytes stimulation test (LST) to *M. leprae*	7. Weak or absent LST
8. Positive lepromin reaction	8. Negative lepromin reaction
9. Production of lymphokines (MIF and MAF) on exposure *M. leprae*	9. Lack of lymphokine production
10. Normal T4/T8 ratio	10. Decreased T4/T8 ratio
11. Proliferation of lymphocytes in the paracortical areas of the lymph nodes	11. Depletion of T-lymphocytes from the paracortical areas, replacement by macrophages
12. Compact granulomatous inflammatory response	12. Loose granuloma
13. Epitheliod cell response with effective phagocytosis with lysis of *M. leprae*	13. Macrophage response with efficient phagocytosis, but ineffective lysis of bacilli
14. T-helper/inducer (T4) cells predominate in tuberculoid granuloma	14. T-suppressor/cytotoxic (T8) cells predominate in lepromatous granuloma
15. T-suppressor/cytotoxic cells form a lymphocytic mantle surrounding the granuloma. T-helper/inducer cells diffusely scattered in the granuloma	15. No such segregation of T-cell subpopulation in lepromatous granuloma
16. Low titers of specific IgG antibodies against *M. leprae*	16. High titers of specific IgG antibodies against *M. leprae*
17. Production of IL-2 by T-cells on exposure to *M. leprae*	17. Failure to produce IL-2
18. Type I (lepra) upgrading or downgrading reaction, an expression of delayed hypersensitivity (gell and coombs type IV reaction)	18. Type II (ENL) reaction, an expression of immune complex reaction (gell and coombs type III reaction)
19. Alteration in lepromin, LTT, cellular changes in paracortical areas of LN, changes in T-cell count, alteration in NK cell activity, elevated levels of IL-2 and IL-2R, during reaction	19. Lowering of C3 and increased C3 d. Circulating immune complexes (CIC). Alteration IgG, IgM during reaction
20. Acute phase reactant may or may not change	20. Increase in C-reactive protein, fibrinogen degradation product, α-antitrypsin and B-2 macroglobulins

▮ RECOMMENDED READING

1. Anonymous. WHO expert committee on leprosy. Fourth Report. WHO Technical Report Series No. 459, 1970.
2. Chiewsilp P, Petchclai B, Chirachariyavej T, Ramasoota T. Immunoglobulins in leprosy. *Int J Lepr Other Mycobact Dis*. 1985;53:28-32.
3. Dharmendra. The active principle of lepromin is a protein antigen of the bacillus. *Lepr India*. 1941; 13:89-103.
4. Fernandez JMM. The early reaction induced by lepromin. *Int J Leprosy*. 1940;8:1-2.
5. Jesudasan K, Christian M, Chacko CJ, Keystone JS. Comparative studies in human and armadillo derived Mitsuda lepromin. *Lepr Rev*. 1985;56:303-308.
6. Mitsuda K. On the value of a skin reaction to suspension of leprosy nodules. *Jpn J Dermatol Urol*. 1919;19:697-708.
7. Narayan RB. Immunopathology of leprosy granulomas--current status: a review. *Lepr Rev*. 1988;59:75-82.
8. Nath I. Immunological aspects of human leprosy. *Lepr India*. 1983;55:752-762.
9. Rea TH, Bakke AC, Parker JW, Modlin RL, Horwitz DA. Peripheral blood T lymphocytes subsets in leprosy. *Int J Lepr Other Mycobact Dis*. 1984;52:311-317.
10. Sehgal VN, Bhattacharya SN, Shah Y, Sharma VK, Gupta CK. Soluble interleukin-2 receptors: levels in leprosy, and during and after type 1 (lepra) and type 2 (ENL) reactions. *Lep Rev*. 1991;62:262-268.
11. Sehgal VN, Joginder, Sharma VK. Immunology of leprosy. A comprehensive survey. *Int J Dermatol*. 1989;28:574-584.

5

Classification of Leprosy

Classification is an effective means of understanding and communicating a difficult disease. Leprosy is a disease with various manifestations and, therefore, difficult to understand without comprehensive classification. The attempts have been made to classify the disease since long, but consensus has never been arrived at. Nevertheless, the basis of classification has been defined time and again. Even though clinical manifestations have been mainly used for classifying leprosy, the bacteriological examination is indispensable. Ideally, immunological and histopathological basis should form a part accompaniment of the classification.

At present the two classification, *Madrid* and *Indian Leprologists'Association Classification* — have been recognized. They are widely used in leprosy centers and in leprosy field work programs.

Madrid classification (1953): This divides leprosy spectrum into two types and two groups which are outlines below:

Lepromatous type (L)
- Macular
- Diffuse
- Infiltrated
- Nodular
- Neuritic, pure (?)

Tuberculoid type (T)
- Macular (Tm)
- Minor tuberculoid [micropapuloid (Tt]
- Major tuberculoid (plaques, annular lesions, etc.) (TT)
- Neuritic, pure (Tn)

Indeterminate (I)
- Macular (Im)
- Neuritic, pure (In)

Borderline [dimorphous groups (B)]
- Infiltrate
- Others (?)

INDIAN LEPROLOGISTS' ASSOCIATION CLASSIFICATION (1955)

This classification too divides leprosy into four types and two groups in contrast to the *Madrid classification*. The subtypes described in Madrid classification do not find a place in this classification. The following are its outlines:
- Lepromatous (L)
- Tuberculoid (T)
- Maculo-anesthetic (MA)
- Polyneuritic (P)
- Borderline (B)
- Indeterminate (I)

On comparison, the above two classifications are essentially the same. Both of these are agreed on tuberculoid, lepromatous and indeterminate leprosy. The difference of opinion rests mainly on the neural cases. The *Indian Leprologists' Classification* has separated and casted them under a separate heading of polyneuritic in which noskin lesions exist. On the other hand, the other one divides pure neural cases into lepromatous (bacteriologically positive) and tuberculoid (bacteriologically negative). Similarly, maculo-anesthetic has been given due importance in *Indian Leprologists' Classification*. However, it seems maculo-anesthetic of *Indian Leprologists' Classification* corresponds to macules of tuberculoid type of *Madrid Classification*. There is hardly anything to choose between the two, the *Indian Leprologists' Classification* may, however, suit the Indian setting.

FIELD WORKERS' CLASSIFICATION

For the leprosy workers working on field projects, leprosy could be classified as tuberculoid, lepromatous, indeterminate and polyneuritic. This classification is comprehensive and useful. Polyneuritic in particular, must form a part component of the same, because this entity is well recognized, especially in Indian subcontinent. In addition, the cases should also be delineated into infectious (open) and noninfectious (closed) type on the basis of bacteriological skin-slit examination. This is of course of considerable help for the purpose of *Leprosy Control Program*. All the bacteriologically positive cases should be grouped as lepromatous (open cases), while other cases as tuberculoid (noninfectious cases). Its outlines are given below:
- Tuberculoid (closed cases)
- Lepromatous (open cases)
- Indeterminate
- Polyneuritic
- Unclassified.

RIDLEY AND JOPLING'S CLASSIFICATION (1966)

This is a recent and widely acclaimed classification and it is useful for research work. It takes into account the immunological and histopathological basis in addition to the clinical and bacteriological findings. The classification divides leprosy into five groups:
- Tuberculoid tuberculoid (TT)
- Borderline tuberculoid (BT)
- Borderline borderline/midborderline (BB)
- Borderline lepromatous (BL)
- Lepromatous lepromatous (LL)

The clinical features of the lesions are easy to understand, for the purpose of delineating then into different groups.

TUBERCULOID TUBERCULOID (TT)

The diagnosis of this group is primarily made on the morphology of the lesions, the number of lesions and the involvement of nerves proximal to or feeding the patch(es). The details of their features are outlined below.

Hypopigmented and/or erythematous macules, plaques, with well-defined erythematous raised border, and a central flattening-saucer the right way up. The lesion usually is bald and dry. There is a complete loss of sensation of temperature, touch and pain. The number of lesion(s) usually varies from 1 to 3. The nerves proximal to or feeding the patches are thickened and/or tender.

Lepromin test is $3+++$.

I Tuberculoid Tuberculoid (TT)
1. Hypopigmented/erythematous macules/plaques
2. Well-defined dry, scaly, indurated Induration marked at the periphery center may show healing/pigmentation
3. Impairment /complete loss of sweating
4. Partial or complete loss of hair
5. Sensations are impaired/lost
6. Number less than 3
7. Thickening or tenderness or both, of nerves feeding/supplying the patch.

BORDERLINE TUBERCULOID (BT)

The diagnosis of this group is based on hypopigmented or erythematous macules or plaques with either well-defined and/or irregular serrated borders. The presence of satellite lesions is contributory. The lesions are usually dry, bald and have impairment of sensations. The numbers of lesions vary from 3 to 10. The finding of thickened and/or tender nerve in the vicinity of the lesion is of considerable assistance.

Lepromin test $1+$ to $2+$.

II Borderline Tuberculoid (BT)

1. Hypopigmented/erythematous macules/plaques with well-defined yet irregular margins
2. Lesions are dry, scaly, induration marked at the periphery
3. Satellite lesions
4. Impairment/complete loss of sweating
5. Partial/total loss of hair
6. Sensations are impaired/totally lost
7. Number less than 10
8. Nerves supplying/feeding the patches thickened or tender or both.

■ BORDERLINE BORDERLINE (BB)

The diagnosis of this group is rather fascinating because it reflects an unstable character of the disease wherein the morphology of the lesion is corresponding to the tuberculoid spectrum of leprosy on the one hand and lepromatous on the other. The essential morphological features of tuberculoid are similar to those described earlier while the features of lepromatous (*vide infra*) are the same as described later. However, the number of lesions resembling the tuberculoid and lepromatous end of the leprosy spectrum is almost equal.

Lepromin test (+) or (–).

III Borderline Borderline (BB)

1. Lesions show morphology of tuberculoid as well as lepromatous HD
2. The number of lesions resembling tuberculoid morphology is almost equal to those resembling lepromatous HD
3. Lesions are bilateral but symmetrical
4. Number of lesions numerous, but countable
5. Nerves thickened or tender or both.

■ BORDERLINE LEPROMATOUS (BL)

This group too has the morphological features similar to borderline borderline. However, the lesions conforming to lepromatous are predominant as compared to tuberculoid morphology. The number

of lesions are numerous, usually uncountable. The tendency of the lesions to be almost symmetrical is another contributory features. Asymmetrical affliction of the nerves in the form of thickening and/or tenderness is helpful in the diagnosis.

Lepromin is negative (–).

IV. Borderline Lepromatous (BL)

1. Lesions show morphology of tuberculoid as well as lepromatous HD
2. Number of lesions resembling lepromatous morphology is much more than those resembling tuberculoid lesions
3. Lesions are bilateral, tending to be symmetrical
4. Number of lesions numerous, and uncountable
5. Nerves may show thickening or tenderness or both.

■ LEPROMATOUS LEPROMATOUS (LL)

The diagnosis of this group is formed by the presence of numerous erythematous, shiny, smooth, macules, papules, nodules, plaques, disposed in an almost bilaterally symmetrical manner. The diffuse infiltration of the skin surface is a helpful diagnostic criterion. The sensations in the lesions are usually preserved. 'Gloves and stocking' type of anesthesia is observed in the later stages of the disease.

Lepromin is negative (–).

V. Lepromatous Lepromatous (LL)

1. Hypopigmented/erythematous macules, plaques, papules/nodules
2. Margins of the macules are hazy and merging imperceptibly into the surrounding skin
3. The lesions are smooth and shiny
4. Usually no impairment of sweating and loss of hair
5. Lesions are bilateral and symmetrical
6. Number of lesions is numerous, uncountable
7. Multiple nerves thickening only in late stages
8. Loss of eyebrows
9. Ears may be infiltrated
10. There may be systemic involvement of liver, spleen, bone marrow, kidneys and testes.

▌RECOMMENDED READING

1. Ridley DS, Jopling WH. Classification of leprosy according to immunity. A five-group system. *Int J Lepr Other Mycobact Dis.* 1966;34:255-273.
2. Ridley DS. Histological classification and the immunological spectrum of leprosy. *Bull World Health Organ.* 1974;51:451-465.
3. Sehgal VN, Jain MK, Srivastava G. Evolution of classification of leprosy. *Int J Dermatol.* 1989;28:161-167.
4. Sehgal VN, Koranne RV, Sehgal S, Beoher PC, Sharma VK. Correlation of morphological, bacteriological, histopathological and immunological features of leprosy. A double-blind study. *J Dermatol.* 1985;12:243-250.
5. Sehgal VN. A seven group classification for institutional and field work. *Lepr Rev.* 1989;60:75.
6. Sehgal VN. Clinical criteria for diagnosis of Hansen's disease. *The Star.* 1990;14:16.

6

Tuberculoid Leprosy

Tuberculoid is a fairly common type of leprosy throughout the world. Its global prevalence is variable, but it forms 60–80 percent of leprosy patients in the Indian subcontinent. It corresponds to tuberculoid of *Madrid and Ridley* and *Jopling's* classifications. It occurs in both males and females. It may affect persons of any age group, but is commonly seen between 20 and 40 years. It is a closed leprosy largely non-infectious—for the lesions are bacteriologically negative by routine slit-skin smear examination.

▮ CLINICAL FEATURES

The patients may present with one or more symptoms-change in the color of the skin, numbness and tingling, impairment or loss of sensations, blisters or ulcers on the hands and feet, weakness and wasting of the muscles, contractures and wrist and foot drop.

The skin, cutaneous and peripheral nerves and the regional lymph nodes are the sites of affliction in tuberculoid leprosy.

Skin lesions: Tuberculoid leprosy may affect any part of the skin surface. The lesions are usually single (Fig 6.1) two or three lesions may be seen (Figs 6.2A to D), but are numerous. The lesion is well-defined, hypopigmented, erythematous dry, scaly and indurated (Figs 6.3 to 6.5). The induration determines the thickness of the lesion and is variable. It is marked at the periphery and

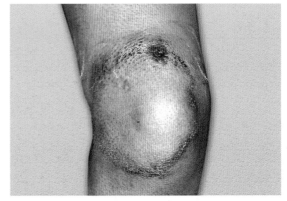

Fig. 6.1: Tuberculoid tuberculoid (TT): A single hypopigmented erythematous, scaly, bald patch with well-defined indurated borders located over the knee joint. The patch is totally anesthetic. The intermediate and medial cutaneous nerves of thigh are thickened and tender. AFB-negative

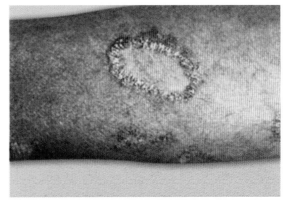

Fig. 6.2A: Tuberculoid tuberculoid (TT): The classical lesion-saucer the right way up

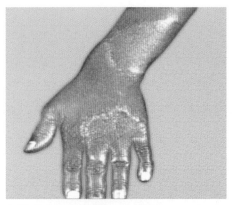

Fig. 6.2B: Tuberculoid tuberculoid lesions on the dorsum of the hand

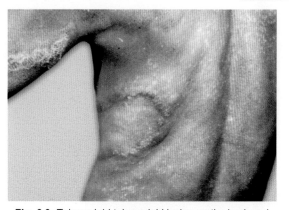

Fig. 6.3: Tuberculoid tuberculoid lesion on the back and upper arm

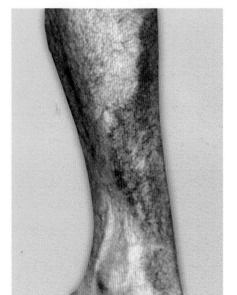

Fig. 6.2C: Tuberculoid tuberculoid lesion on the hand

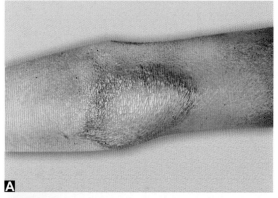

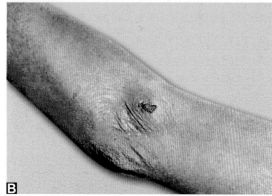

Figs 6.4A and B: Tuberculoid tuberculoid (TT): Depicting marked atrophy of the lesions

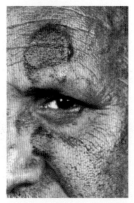

Fig. 6.2D: Tuberculoid tuberculoid lesion on the forehead

is sloping toward the center of the lesion giving an appearance a *saucer right way up* (Figs 6.6 and 6.7). They are bald due to complete or partial loss of hairs.

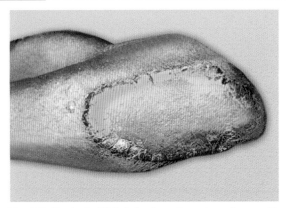

Fig. 6.5: Psoriasis: Well-defined, erythematous plaque with silvery white, micaceous scales situated over the elbow and the extensor aspect. Auspitz sign positive. Sensation intact

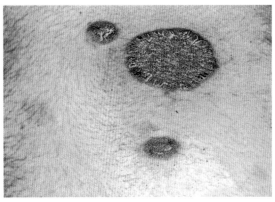

Fig. 6.6: Psoriasis: Well-defined, erythemato-scaly lesion over the back. Auspitz sign positive. Sensations intact

Sensations: Impairment or complete loss of sensation of the lesion is a cardinal feature. It is usually preceded by numbness and tingling. There is impairment or loss of temperature, light and pain in that sequence.

Nerves: Thickening and/or tenderness of the cutaneous and peripheral nerves is another cardinal sign. It is only the regional nerves, supplying or feeding the patch, which are affected. At times, localized swellings along the nerve—the nerve abscess—may be present.

Bacteriology: Day-to-day slit-skin smear for *Mycobacterium leprae* is usually negative.

Lepromin reaction: The lepromin reaction is always strongly positive $(+++)$.

VARIANTS

In addition to the clinical features recounted above, certain variations in the lesions may also be seen. Hypopigmentation is usual; however, at times hyperpigmentation may be seen at the center of the lesion (Figs 6.8 and 6.9). Similarly, an atrophy or scar may be present (Figs 6.10 and 6.11).

Tuberculoid major: In this variety, the lesions are grossly thickened, and elevated. The thickening may be uniform or confined to the periphery with a depressed center. Hence, the margin is well-defined and stands out clearly (Figs 6.12A and B). The surface may be smooth or scaly.

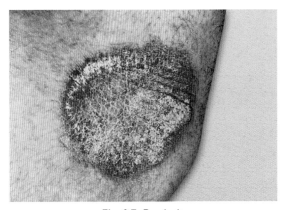

Fig. 6.7: Psoriasis

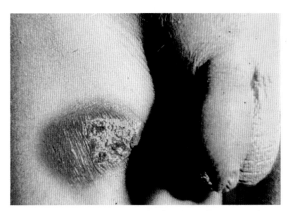

Fig. 6.8: Lupus vulgaris: Well-defined, erythematous, indurated plaque with advancing margins. Atrophy of the skin is conspicuous, suggesting healing at places

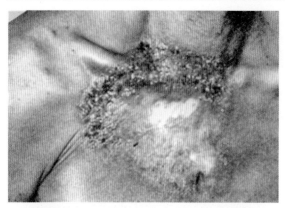

Fig. 6.9: Lupus vulgaris: Lesions on front of the chest

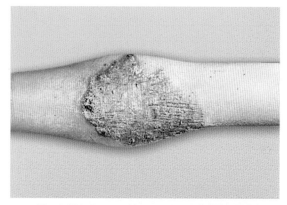

Fig. 6.12A: Lupus vulgaris: Near the elbow joint

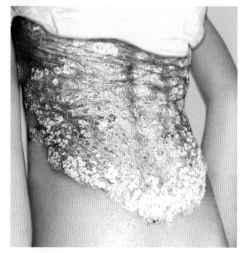

Fig. 6.10: Lupus vulgaris: On the back

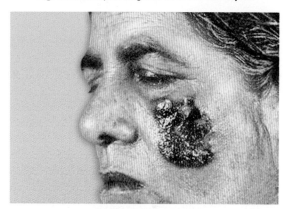

Fig. 6.12B: Lupus vulgaris: Lesions on the face

Tuberculoid minor: In this variety, the lesions are slightly or moderately raised. The induration is confined to the margin or to a part of the margin with a flat hypopigmented or normal colored center (Fig. 6.13)

DIAGNOSIS

It is based on the cardinal clinical features—the morphology of the lesions, thickening and/or tenderness of the cutaneous and peripheral regional nerves, impairment or loss of sensation of temperature, touch and pain in skin lesions, and also in the peripheral part of the limbs. The diagnosis is established by the sweat test demonstrating sweat response in the patch (Fig. 6.14) and by salient histological features. The details of sweat test are given below.

Sweat test: 0.1 ml (0.025 mg) of carbachol (carba-minyol choline) is injected into the hypopigmented

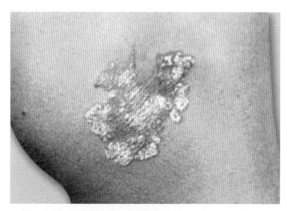

Fig. 6.11: Lupus vulgaris: Showing marked atrophy at places

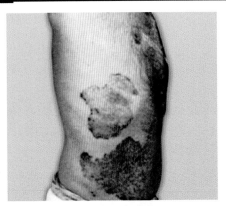

Fig. 6.13: Tinea circinata: Well-defined, intensely itchy erythemato-scaly lesions spreading at the periphery and clearing at the center. KOH positive

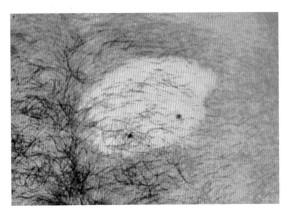

Fig. 6.14: Nevus anamicus: Well-circumscribed, hypopigmented macule over the abdomen. Hair and sensations are well preserved. Vascular response absent on stroking the skin

patch (initial) intradermally, and the area is left covered with Whatman No. 1 filter paper strip impregnated with a 1 percent alcoholic solution of bromophenol blue. The paper is removed after five minutes and the number of blue dots indicative of sweat response should be counted per square inch area around the site of injection. The central smudge at the site of injection is omitted from the count. The results are expressed as under.

0–10 spots	Nil
11–100 spots	+
101–200 spots	+ +
201–300 spots	+ + +
more than 300 spots or large smudge of sweat	+ + + +

Contralateral normal side is used as control. There is either an impairment or complete loss of sweating in the patch.

◼ DIFFERENTIAL DIAGNOSIS

Although, there is hardly any difficulty in making a diagnosis of tuberculoid leprosy, yet there are certain dermatoses which may mislead. The following common conditions with their salient clinical features may assist in differentiating them from tuberculoid leprosy.

Vitiligo: It involves depigmentation of the skin characterized by ivory white macules, flushed to the surface with hyperpigmented margins (Figs 6.15A and B). There is neither impairment nor loss of

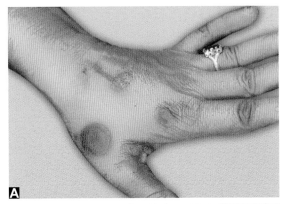

A

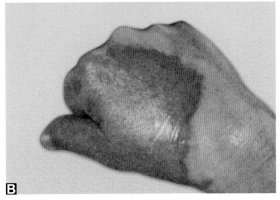

B

Figs 6.15A and B: Granuloma annulare: Well-circumscribed annular, non-scaly plaque with elevated borders over the dorsum of the hand. Sensations intact. Microscopic pathology confirmatory

sensation nor loss of sweating. There is no loss of hair infact leukotrichia may be present.

Tinea corporis: This usually starts as an erythematous, itchy papule which progresses to form a circinate lesion. It is studded at the periphery with papules or papulovesicles. The lesions are scaly, showing clear or apparently normal looking centers (Figs 6.16A and B). They show seasonal variations—common in hot and humid climate. The demonstration of fungus in 10 percent KOH from the scrapings seen under the microscope and their recovery in saboraud agar medium is confirmatory.

Pityriasis versicolor: It is characterized by asymptomatic, hypopigmented, mildly scaly,

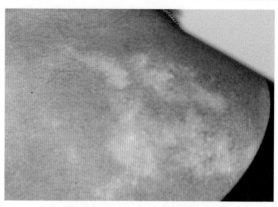
Fig. 6.17: Pitriasis Versicolor on the back

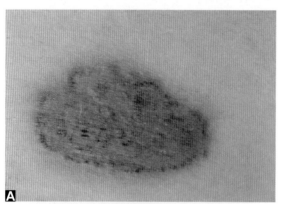
A

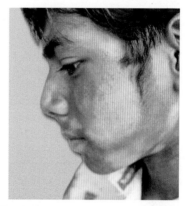
Fig. 6.18: Pityriasis simplex over the face

multiple macules distributed on the body surface, largely corresponding to the 'lady's bathing suit' (Fig. 6.17). Seasonal variation is its main feature. The diagnosis could confirm by finding of mycelia and spores of *Malassezia furfur* in the scrapings seen under the microscope.

Pityriasis simplex: It is clinically recognized as ill-defined, hypopigmented, asymptomatic macules usually located on the face amongst children (Fig. 6.18). The condition is transitory and occurs in malnourished persons. It is a subliminal infection of the skin, due to *Staphylococcus*. The absence of cardinal clinical features of leprosy helps in its exclusion.

Circinate syphilides: This condition sometimes creates a problem in diagnosis of tuberculoid leprosy. However, history of sexual exposure, primary chancre

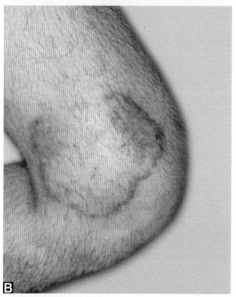
B
Figs 6.16A and B: Tinea corporis a and b

or scar on the genitals and polymorphic syphilitic rash renders the help in diagnosis (Fig. 6.19). The diagnosis may be confirmed by the demonstration of *Treponema pallidum* in the lesion and reaction serological test for syphilis.

Psoriasis: The lesions of this condition are typical—they are erythemato-scaly eruptions, single or multiple, disposed primarily on the extensor surfaces of the body. The scales are lamellated and silvery white (Figs 6.20A and B). Auspitz's sign is positive, evident as a pinpoint bleeding on grattage. Histology is diagnostic.

Pityriasis rosea: It is characterized by appearance of multiple, oval, well-defined, erythematous, scaly eruptions, disposed along the body cleavages tree (Fig 6.21). The condition is asymptomatic and self-limiting. The initial lesion—a herald patch—is diagnostic hallmark of the disease.

Naevus anaemicus: It is a birthmark and it may appear at the time of birth, during childhood or at puberty. It is an ill-defined, hypopigmented macule, wherein the vascular response is lacking due to the absence of blood vessels. Its diagnosis is excluded by the absence of cardinal clinical features of tuberculoid leprosy. On diascopic examination, it is indistinguishable from the surrounding skin (Fig. 6.22).

Discoid lupus erythematosus: It is a fascinating condition which manifests as erythematous, scaly macules the scales being located at the hair follicles. Atrophy in the lesion is seen with the progression of the condition (Fig. 6.23). It affects the butterfly area of the face, the forehead, ears and upper chest. The histology of the lesion is confirmatory.

Morphea: It starts as an indurated, oval or round plaque of lilac or dark red color. The skin becomes

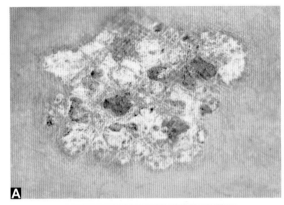

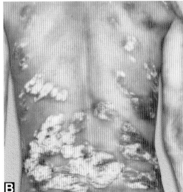

Figs 6.20A and B: Psoriasis plaque depicting silvery white, dry brittle scales

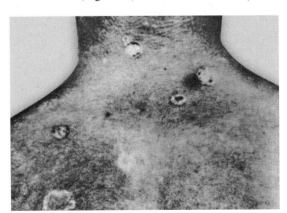

Fig. 6.19: Circinata syphilides over the side of the neck

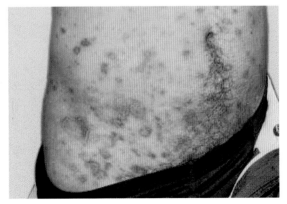

Fig. 6.21: Pityriasis rosea over the lower chest and upper abdomen

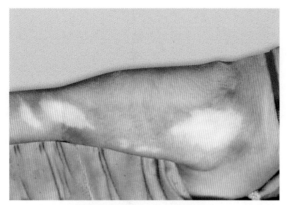

Fig. 6.22: Neavus anaemicus

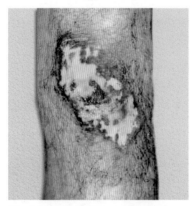

Fig. 6.23: Discoid lupus erythematosus

atrophic, ivory white, in due course. The course of the lesion is marked by spontaneous remission, residual pigmentation and atrophy. Absence of cardinal clinical signs of leprosy and characterized histopathology of the lesion is diagnostic of the condition.

Table 6.1: Chemotherapy for paucibacillary (PB) leprosy

Clinical group	Drugs	Dosage and Mode of administration	Duration
1*, TT	Rifampicin	600 mg once monthly supervised	6 doses rifampicin to be administered in maximum of nine months
	Dapsone	100 mg daily self-administered	

TREATMENT

Tuberculoid leprosy should be treated by recommended standard regimen for paucibacillary (PB) leprosy. The standard regimen is formed by 600 mg of rifampicin once a month for 6 months plus diaminodiphenyl sulfone 100 mg (1–2 mg/kg body weight) daily for 6 months. The administration of rifampicin should be supervised, while dapsone may be taken by the patient himself. The therapy is considered adequate if 6 doses of rifampicin are given, atleast 4 weeks apart, within a total of 9 months. If the treatment is interrupted, the regimen should be commenced where it was left off, to complete the full course (Table 6.1).

RECOMMENDED READING

1. Parikh AC, Ganpati R, Kapadia BI, Naik SS. Acetylcholine test for anhydrosis in leprosy. *Lepr Rev*. 1966;37:231-237.
2. Yawalkar SJ, Sanjana HB. Effect of DDS therapy on the acetylcholine sweat function test in fifty cases of tuberculoid and maculoanesthetic leprosy. *Int J Lepr Other Mycobact Dis*. 1974;42:55-57.

Maculo-anesthetic Leprosy

Maculo-anesthetic leprosy is similar to macule of tuberculoid leprosy of *Madrid Classification*. It is well recognized entity in the Indian subcontinent. It is closed leprosy, largely non-infectious, for bacilli are difficult to demonstrate by slit-skin smear examination. It is seen both in males and females, but is common in the younger age group, especially children.

◼ CLINICAL FEATURES

Usually the patient reports with discoloration over the skin. Numbness, tingling and impairment or loss of sensation occurs in the patch or the peripheral portion of the extremities. It affects the skin surface, and also the regional cutaneous and peripheral nerves.

Skin lesion: These are characterized by well-defined, hypopigmented, flat; macules which are flushed to the skin surface (Figs 7.1 to 7.3). Erythema may be an associated presenting feature. They are usually single or a few, but never scaly with partial or complete loss of hairs. Impairment or loss of sweating may be an associated clinical manifestation.

Sensations: There may be hypoaesthesia or anesthesia. The sensation of temperature, fine touch and pain may be affected in that sequence.

Nerves: The affliction of the cutaneous and/or peripheral nerves may be an associated feature. The regional nerves supplying or feeding the patch(es) may be moderately thickened and/or tender.

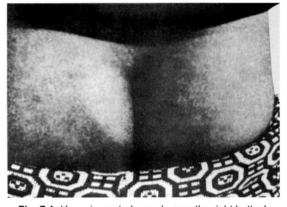
Fig. 7.1: Hypopigmented macule over the right buttock

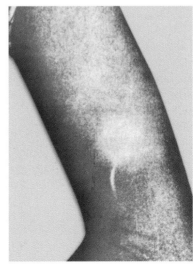
Fig. 7.2: Hypopigmented macule over the upper arm

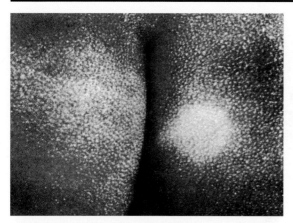

Fig. 7.3: Well-defined hypopigmented macule of maculo-anesthetic leprosy

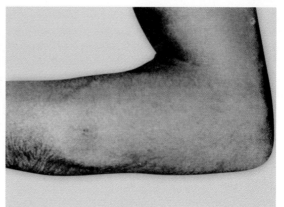

Fig. 7.4

Bacteriology: The routine slit-skin smear examination for lepra bacilli is negative.

Lepromin test: It is usually moderately to strongly positive.

Variants

Usually a single macule is seen, but multiple lesions may at times be present. Similarly, the lesions are usually of small size, occasionally, moderate or very big macule may be the presenting feature. Hypopigmentation is the rule; sometimes hyperpigmentation is also seen (Figs 7.4 and 7.5). At times, atrophy in the center of the lesion may be a feature.

Diagnosis

In addition to the morphology of the skin lesions, disturbance of sensations, thickening and/or tenderness of the regional nerves are diagnostic clinical features. Furthermore, induration is conspicuous by its absence in maculo-anesthetic leprosy.

Impairment or complete loss of sweating is an important diagnostic test, the details of which have already been discussed under the diagnosis of 'tuberculoid leprosy'. Histology of the lesions may be contributory.

Differential Diagnosis

The following conditions with their salient features may be considered in the differential diagnosis.

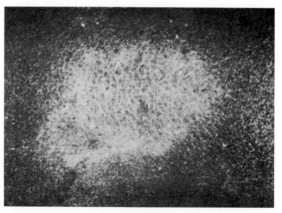

Fig. 7.5

Figs 7.4 and 7.5: Well-defined macule with hyperpigmentation at the centre

Nevus anemicus: It is a birth mark; it may appear at the time of birth, during childhood or at puberty. It is an ill-defined, hypopigmented macule, wherein the vascular response is lacking due to absence of clinical features of maculo-anesthetic leprosy described earlier. On diascopic examination, it is indistinguishable from the surrounding skin.

Pityriasis simplex: It is clinically recognized as ill-defined, hypopigmented, asymptomatic macules usually located on the face, amongst children. The condition is transitory, and occurs in malnourished persons. It is subliminal infection of the skin due to *Staphylococcus*. The absence of cardinal clinical features of leprosy helps in its exclusion.

Pityriasis versicolor: It is characterized by asymptomatic, hypopigmented, mildly scaly, multiple macules, distributed on the body surface, corresponding largely to the 'lady's bathing suit'. Seasonal variation is its feature. The diagnosis is confirmed by finding mycelia and spores of *Malassezia furfur* when the scraping is seen under the microscope.

Morphea: This starts as an indurated, oval or round plaque of lilac or dark red color. The skin becomes atrophic, ivory white, in due course. The course of the lesion is marked by spontaneous remission, residual pigmentation, and atrophy. Absence of cardinal clinical signs of leprosy and characteristic histopathology of the lesion is diagnostic of the condition.

Pre-vitiligo: It is the initial stage of vitiligo wherein there is an insidious loss of pigmentation of the skin. The lesions are hypopigmented and ill-defined. They may progress to form ivory white macules—classical lesions of vitiligo. There is no loss of hair or sweating or disturbance of sensations. Thickening and/or tenderness of the regional nerves is lacking.

Post-inflammatory hypopigmentation: The lesions are hypopigmented with ill-defined margins. They are the remnants of various inflammatory dermatoses. The history of an inflammatory dermatosis is affirmative and of course, conspicuous absence of characteristic clinical features of maculo-anesthetic leprosy is helpful.

▌TREATMENT

Maculo-anesthetic leprosy should be treated in a similar fashion as that of tuberculoid (paucibacillary), the details of which are described earlier (see table 6.1).

▌RECOMMENDED READING

1. Wade HW. Maculo-anaesthetic leprosy, classification. *Int J Lepr.* 1952;20:444.

Lepromatous Leprosy

Lepromatous leprosy is a severe manifestation of leprosy. Its global prevalence is variable, being 10–20 percent in Indian subcontinent. It corresponds to lepromatous leprosy of *Madrid* and *Ridley* and *Jopling's* classifications. It affects both males and females of all age groups, but frequently seen between 20 and 59 years.

CLINICAL FEATURES

In this disease the patient may present with different symptoms such as various skin changes, bleeding from the nose, hoarseness of voice, numbness and tingling in the limbs, blisters, ulcers and other trophic changes like weakness, wasting, contractures of muscles and wrist or foot drops. The skin changes are striking and instantly attract the clinician's attention.

It is a generalized disease affecting the skin, mucous membranes, nerves and the reticuloendothelial system. Largely, the systemic involvements are asymptomatic, except that of tests.

Skin lesions: They start as multiple, hypopigmented, smooth, erythematous macules. They are generalized and bilaterally symmetrical. The outline of the macules is hazy, merging imperceptibly with the surrounding skin. There is an increasing induration with the progress of the disease. The indurated macules may later coalesce to form large plaque. The skin becomes smooth and shiny. The whole or any part of the skin surface may be affected, but the involvement of the face is prominent. Thickening of the ear lobes and loss of eyebrows are a cardinal manifestation (Figs 8.1 to 8.16), as is supracilliary madaroses.

Sensation: The modalities of sensation are usually unaffected in the early stages.

Blunting of sensations may, however, be seen in grossly indurated lesions.

Nerves: There is involvement of multiple nerves, but the cardinal feature of tenderness is usually lacking.

Bacteriological examination: Slit-skin smears from the affected sites are strongly positive (+ + +) for the bacilli.

Lepromin test: It is always negative.

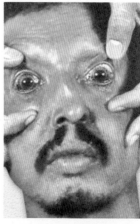

Fig. 8.1: Lepromatous leprosy depicting pigmentation after clofazimine therapy

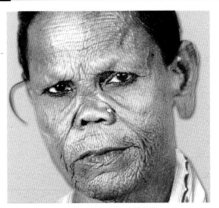

Fig. 8.2: Lepromatous leprosy: A conspicuous facial appearance characterized by marked depression of the bridge of the nose, superciliary madarosis and marked wrinkling of the face, indicating grade II deformity

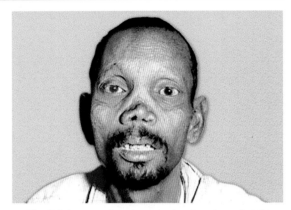

Fig. 8.5: Lepromatous leprosy showing characteristic deformity of the nose

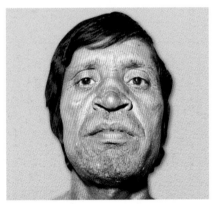

Fig. 8.3: Lepromatous leprosy: Diffuse erythematous infiltration over the face giving it a shiny appearance. Ciliary and superciliary madarosis with depression of bridge of nose

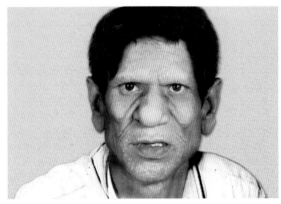

Fig. 8.6: Lepromatous leprosy demonstrating shiny, wrinkled face with ciliary and superciliary madarosis

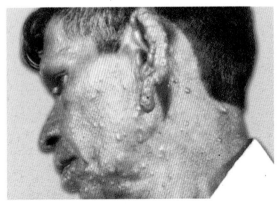

Fig. 8.4: Lepromatous leprosy: Multiple, nodular lesions of varying sizes located over the erythematous, diffuse infilteration over the face and left ear

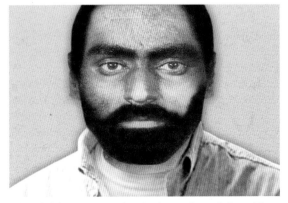

Fig. 8.7: Lepromatous leprosy hyperpigmentation of the face following clofazmine therapy

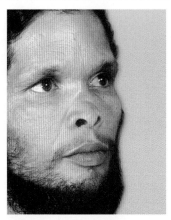

Fig. 8.8: Lepromatous leprosy showing depression of the bridge of nose and slight madarosis

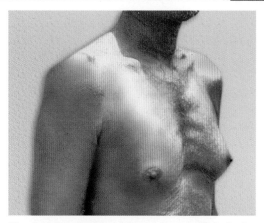

Fig. 8.11: Lepromatous leprosy: A case with testicular atrophy gynecomastia-type I disability

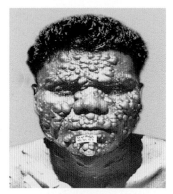

Fig. 8.9: Lepromatous leprosy: Documenting multiple nodules of different sizes over the face

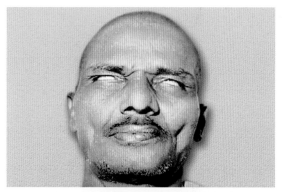

Fig. 8.12: Lepromatous leprosy: Bilaterally symmetrical infracuclear facial paisy showing lagophthalmos

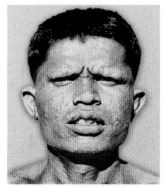

Fig. 8.10: Lepromatous leprosy: Diffuse infiltration of the face with ciliary and supercilary madarosis

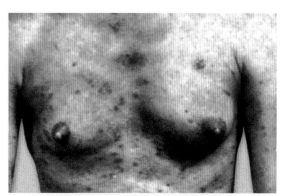

Fig. 8.13: Lepromatous leprosy: A case with testicular atrophy showing gynecomastia

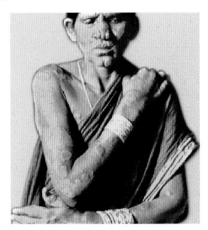

Fig. 8.14: Lepromatous leprosy showing markedly indurated lesions

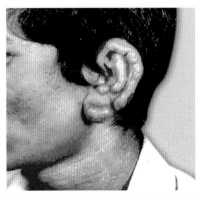

Fig. 8.15: Lepromatous leprosy showing nodular infiltration of the ear

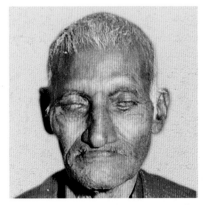

Fig. 8.16: Lepromatous leprosy showing bilateral lagophthalmos

Variants

The indurations (infiltration) of the skin is a cardinal sign of lepromatous leprosy. The degree and extend of the induration determines the morphological features of the lesions. Hence, it may present as nodules, ulcerative, noduloulcerative and diffuse infiltrative lesions.

Nodules: Gross, localized induration of the lesions leads to formation of subcutaneous mobile nodules. The size of these lesions is variable. They may be a few or multiple. They may appear anywhere on the body, the face, and the ear lobes being the common sites of involvement. Marked induration of the face with multiple superimposed nodules—leonine facies—is a classic presentation.

Ulcers: These may occur over the indurated or nodular lesions. The nodules may in the late stages become fixed to the skin and form ulcers. They may be single or multiple and distributed on any part of the body. The crops of nodules slowly progress to form multiple ulcers Lucio's phenomenon—seen in some parts of the world, especially Mexico.

Diffuse infiltration: Another variant is the diffuse infiltration of the skin. It is slowly progressive induration, which may cover a part or whole of the skin surface. The skin is considerably thickened and unevenly indurated. It becomes erythematous, shiny and smooth. There is complete loss of hair and the pilosebaceous orifices may become prominent.

Histoid leprosy: This variant of leprosy develops in long standing advanced cases of multibacillary leprosy. It is characterized by formation of subcutaneous nodules of varying sizes. These nodules may remain subcutaneous for a long period in many cases. They tend to migrate toward the skin surface to fuse with the dermis. They may later unite to form elevated protuberant masses (Figs 8.17A to E). Sometimes, however, the nodules may be superficial, and may become protuberant and even pedunculated. The bacteriological finding is the most striking distinguishing feature in the lesions. The bacilli are abundant and regular staining, but the formation of globi is conspicuous by its absence.

Mucous membranes: Involvement of the mucous membranes is frequent. The mucous membranes of the upper respiratory tract comprising nasal,

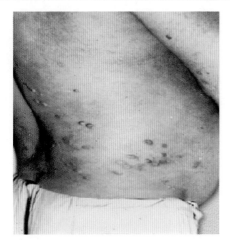

Fig. 8.17A: Shows lesions in back

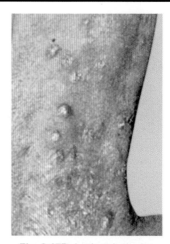

Fig. 8.17D: Lesions in the leg

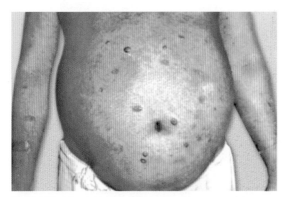

Fig. 8.17B: Histoid leprosy: Shiny translucent nodules over the abdomen

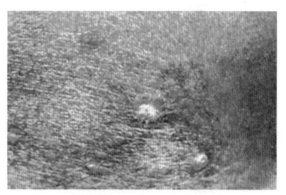

Fig. 8.17E: Lesions on the back

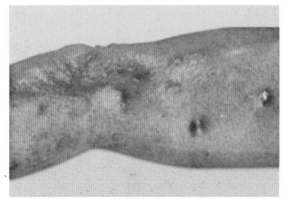

Fig. 8.17C: Lesions over the upper arm and forearm

nasopharyngeal and laryngeal mucosae are the sites of affliction.

Nasal mucosa: Nasal stuffiness is the earliest sign of involvement of nasal mucosa. It is because of inflammation of the mucous membranes. It may gradually progress to form small, grayish-white indurated lesions, which may soon break to form ulcers, giving rise to recurrent bleeding from the nose. Side by side, the cartilaginous part of the nasal septum may be affected causing its necrosis, and nasal deformity—depressed nose—a classical presentation of lepromatous leprosy. Healing by fibrosis may further add to the deformity.

Oropharyngeal mucosa: Similarly, the mucosa of the oral and pharyngeal cavity may be affected. The morphology of the lesions is similar to that described in the preceding paragraph. The extensive involvement of mucous membrane and cartilage of the palate may cause its perforation with symptoms of regurgitation.

Laryngeal mucosa: The mucous membrane of the larynx is affected. It may cause a slowly progressive induration extending to involve its cartilages. The lesions may ulcerate to form painful ulcers. Sometimes it may lead to obstruction and difficult breathing. The vocal cords may similarly be affected, and may cause hoarseness of voice.

Mucous membrane of the eye: Eye may be affected causing conjunctivitis and episcleral nodules, the details of which are described in 'ocular leprosy'.

Systemic involvement: Various organs of the body, viz. liver, spleen, bone marrow and kidney may be affected. Their involvement is largely asymptomatic. The affection of the testis may cause orchitis, resulting in depletion of male hormones. Under such conditions, uni- or bilateral gynecomastia may be a cardinal manifestation.

Diagnosis

The diagnosis is based on the cardinal clinical features, namely the various morphological lesions of the skin, enlargement of the peripheral nerves, and the demonstration of bacilli by slit-skin smears, the latter being strongly positive. Further confirmation is done by the characteristic histopathology.

Differential Diagnosis

The macules of lepromatous leprosy may be required to be differentiated from tuberculoid and maculo-anesthetic leprosy, in addition to previtiligo, pityriasis simplex, nevus anemicus postinflammatory hypopigmentation, morphea, pityriasis rosea, and pityriasis versicolor. The salient clinical features of the later conditions have been outlined in the preceding clinical features, especially of tuberculoid and maculo-anesthetic leprosy.

Tuberculoid leprosy: It is recognized by well-defined hypopigmented, erythematous, dry, scaly and indurated lesions. The center of the lesions is atrophic or apparently normal. Classically, it resembles a 'saucer right way up'. Furthermore, the number of lesions is an important diagnostic parameter. Solitary, two or three lesions are usual. The presence of numerous lesions excludes its diagnosis. Hypoesthesia or anesthesia in the lesions and the peripheral parts of the extremities, along with enlargement and/or tenderness of regional and the peripheral nerves are the cardinal features. Slit-skin smears are, however, negative, Lepromin test is strongly positive (+ + +).

Maculo-anesthetic leprosy: It is characterized by well-defined, hypopigmented, flat macules, which are flushed to the skin surface. The macules are usually single or few, but never numerous. They are dry and scaly with partial or complete loss of hair. Impairment or loss of sweating may be an associated finding. Hypoesthesia or anesthesia may also be a feature. The lesions are bacteriologically negative. Lepromin test is moderately (+) to strongly positive (+ + +).

The diagnosis of well-formed indurated and nodular lesions is hardly difficult. Some cases may, however, pose a problem and may be required to be differentiated from conditions like dermal Leishmaniasis, tertiary yaws, erythema nodosum and neurofibromatosis.

Dermal Leishmaniasis: The formation of multiple nodules is an important clinical feature in an advanced case of dermal Leishmaniasis. The nodules may be generalized or predominantly distributed on the face and the ears like that is lepromatous leprosy (Figs 8.17F to 8.18). But absence of lepra bacilli and the presence of Leishmania Donovani (LD) bodies serve to differentiate from lepromatous leprosy.

Tertiary yaws: Nodular/noduloulcerative lesions characterize the condition. They usually start as multiple, indurated, nontender, mobile, sub-or intracutaneous nodules. The superficial nodules may ulcerate to form crusted discoid or serpiginous ulcers, while the deeper nodules may ulcerate to form clear-cut, large destructive ulcers with dirty yellow slough. They may involve the bone underneath to form destructive bony lesions, the classical being-gangosa with through and through perforation of the face. History of residence in an endemic area, contact with an infected case, remnant skin lesions of early yaws, and absence of cardinal clinical features of leprosy is contributory.

Erythema nodosum: It is a symptom complex, Multiple, transitory erythematous, tender are its clinical features. Their distribution, though generalized, has special predilection for extensor surfaces of the extremities. Remissions and exacerbation is its hallmark. Exclusion of the condition is based on the absence of cardinal signs of leprosy.

Neurofibromatosis

Occasionally, it may cause a diagnostic problem. However, its clinical features are distinct from leprosy. Asymptomatic multiple, soft subcutaneous nodules with pigmented macules-café-au-lait spots, form its clinical features (Figs 8.19A and B). It is progressive, and starts usually in childhood. The involvement of the nerves in the form of swelling

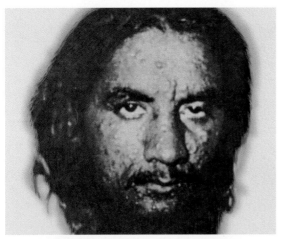

Fig. 8.17F: Dermal leishmaniasis (post-kala azar dermal leishmaniasis: nodular lesions on the face)

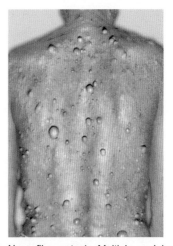

Fig. 8.19A: Neurofibromatosis: Multiple, nodular lesions in the back

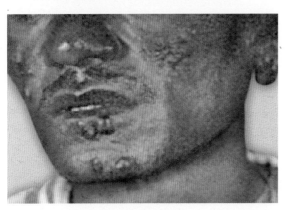

Fig. 8.18: Lepromatous leprosy with nodular lesions on the face. AFB strongly positive

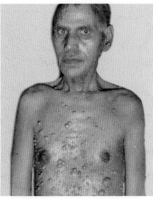

Fig. 8.19B: Neurofibromatosis lesions on front of the trunk

Table 8.1: Chemotherapy for multi-bacillary (MB) leprosy

Clinical type	Drugs	Dosage and Mode of administration	Duration
BT, BB, BL, LL	Rifampicin	600 mg once monthly supervised	2 years or preferably till smear negativity
	Dapsone	100 mg daily self-administered	
	Clofazimine	300 mg supervised every month and 50 mg daily self-administered	

may be an interesting feature. Exclusion of the condition is by its characteristic histology.

TREATMENT

Lepromatous leprosy (multi-bacillary) should be maintained on a multidrug regimen consisting of rifampicin (600 mg once monthly, supervised), clofazimine (300 mg once monthly, supervised, and 50 mg daily self-administered) and diaminodiphenyl sulfone (100 mg daily self-administered) for 2 years or until they become smear negative (Table 8.1). Clinical and bacteriological surveillance after completion of treatment is an important adjuvant. It is, therefore, imperative to examine these cases both clinically and bacteriologically at least once a year for a minimum of 5 years.

RECOMMENDED READING

1. Sehgal VN. Clinical criteria for the diagnosis of Hansen's disease. *The Star*. 1990;14:16.

9

Histoid Leprosy

Histoid leprosy is a peculiar, relatively stable, distinct clinical, bacteriological and histopathological expression of multibacillary leprosy and its exact pathogenesis still remain elusive. It is known to occur in patients on diaminodiphenyl sulfone (DDS) monotherapy for a long time that show initial improvement followed by relapse. Irregular and inadequate therapy may facilitate its occurrence. It is reported in patients who develop secondary drug resistance to DDS. Treatment with DDS alone may create a selective environment, by killing the drug-sensitive microorganisms, which may allow the growth of resistant bacilli. Apart from occurring in patients on DDS monotherapy, it may also arise *de novo*. Augmented cell-mediated immunity is cardinal, and may explain its attempted focalization of lesions.

CLINICAL FEATURES

Histoid leprosy presents in the form of cutaneous, subcutaneous nodules, and/or plaques arising apparently over the normal skin. The cutaneous lesions are firm, reddish or skin colored, dome shaped or oval papules or nodules, regular in contour with shiny and stretched overlying skin and, at times, with a constriction around their bases. The subcutaneous lesions are also common and vary in size, from the smallest that can be palpated to the largest of about 5 cm in diameter. The smaller lesions are soft, whereas, the older and larger nodules are firm and fibrotic. Such nodules may

remain subcutaneous indefinitely or migrate toward the surface and fuse with the dermis, and become elevated and protuberant (Figs 9.1 to 9.3). They may also breakdown to form raw-surfaced lesions. Occasionally, histoid leprosy may manifest as plaques. They are thick scaling pads which usually develop at pressure points. These plaques are sharply delineated. The number of lesions usually varies between 6 and 50. They are usually located over the lower back, buttocks, face, extremities and the bony prominence such as knees and elbows. On the face, the lesions are most prominent over the middle of forehead, cheeks, tip of the nose and chin. The earlobes are infrequently affected, and the loss of eyebrows is unusual. The mucosal surfaces may be affected, and nodules may be encountered

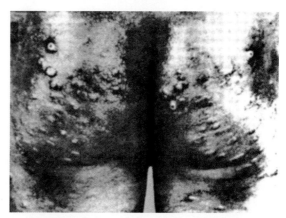

Fig. 9.1: Cutaneous papulonodular lesions over the buttocks; a few healing ulcerated nodules are also seen

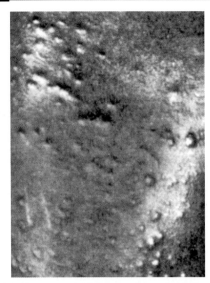

Fig. 9.2: Numerous cutaneous nodules studded over the back

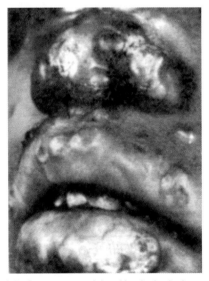

Fig. 9.3: Cutaneous nodules: Hemispherical, smooth, shiny and translucent, a few showing ulceration

on the roof of the mouth, middle of the hard palate and the glans penis. Nasal mucosa may be affected; however, there is no destruction of the nasal cartilage. ENL reaction is uncommon.

Slit-skin Smears

Slit-skin smear examination of the histoid lesion reveals abundance of uniformly staining acid-fast

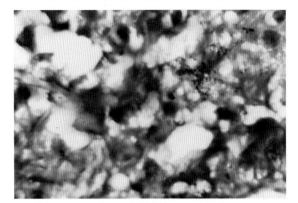

Fig. 9.4: A slit-skin smear of a characteristic plaque (ZN x 100)

leprosy bacilli occurrence singly or in parallel clumps. The bacilli are long with tapering ends as compared with ordinary leprosy bacilli (Fig. 9.4). In contrast, the surrounding, apparently normal skin reveals scant bacilli. Thus, there is a marked discrepancy in the BI from the histoid nodule and the surrounding skin.

Histopathology

Hematoxylin-eosin stained sections from the histoid nodule may be marked by the presence of the lesion in the dermis or subcutaneous tissue or both, a psueudocapsule surrounding the lesion, formed by the compression of the adjacent tissue due to the expanding lesion, conspicuous absence of appendages within the nodule, the presence of numerous, thin spindle-shaped histiocytes arranged either in an intertwining, crisscross or in a whorled fashion, (Figs 9.5, 9.6A and B) and Fite's staining reveals an abundance of AFB within the spindle-shaped cells. They are uniformly staining measurably longer than the ordinary lepra bacilli. They conform to the shape of the histiocytes. They are arranged in groups or parallel bundles along the long axis of the cell. Globi are conspicuously absent.

Cytopathology

Fine-needle aspiration or cytopuncture of skin nodules of histoid leprosy yields cellular aspirates, comprise of cohesive aggregates of spindle shaped macrophages with intracytoplasmic negative images of solid *M. leprae*. Many extracellular negative

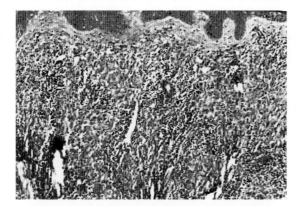

Fig. 9.5: A hypercellular histoid lesion, composed chiefly of fusiform and polygonal histiocytes (H & E x 100)

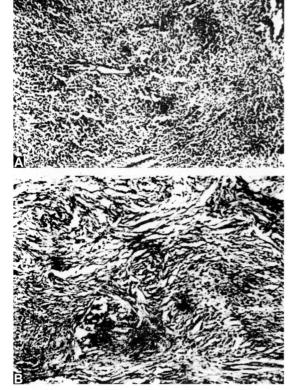

Figs 9.6A and B: Spindle-shaped histiocytes arranged in crisscross/intertwine parallel and whirlwind pattern (H & E x 100)

images may also be seen in the background. Acid-fast stain is positive and demonstrates solid uniform staining, long bacilli displaying the characteristic

histoid habitus. Negative images have also been described in other Mycobacterial diseases, therefore, the diagnosis on fine needle aspiration is only circumstantial and may largely relie on clinico-pathologic correlation.

Histopathology: The microscopic pathology of histoid leprosy evolves with time and is altered by therapy. Many of the salient histopathologic features are based on examination of architectural patterns of the cellular proliferation at low magnification. It is, therefore, imperative to take a biopsy of the entire lesion early in its evolution, and before the administration of the multidrug therapy (MDT). Examination of the sections at scanning magnification is paramount to precisely interpret the micro-scopic pathology. Accordingly, the lesion(s) are circumscribed, cellular, and comprised of interlacing fascicles of spindle-shaped cells, thus, resembling a fibrohistiocytic lesion or dermatofibroma. A narrow Grenz zone is conspicuous just beneath an atrophic epidermis. At the periphery the lesion appears expansile: notwithstanding the few hair follicles entrapped within the proliferating spindle cells, the pilosebaceus units and eccrine glands appear to be pushed outward. However, at higher magnification the spindle cells nature of the lesional cells is apparent. It is not unusual to locate a few foci of chronic inflammatory cells in the sections, Furthermore, the storiform pattern, the spoke-wheel like arrangement of the interlacing bundles of spindle cells, that may be pronounced in some lesions is contributory to the resemblance to fibrohistiocytic tumors. Hyperplasia of the overlying epidermis, sometimes in pseudocarcinomatous proportions, or occasionally a basaloid proliferation resembling basal cell carcinoma may be seen overlying a fibrous histiocytoma. However, epidermal atrophy is the rule of thumb in histoid leprosy, a feature that may assist in forming the diagnosis of the entity. When the cells are examined at high magnification many needle-like intracytoplasmic, negative staining images are seen. These negative images represent *M. lepre* and, when correctly recognized, are clues to the diagnosis. Stain for acid-fast bacilli (Fig. 9.5) reveals numerous organisms corresponding to the negative images. Examination of the tissue outside the periphery of a histoid lesion frequently reveals

Table 9.1: Recommended dose schedule

Drugs	Dose	Duration
1. Diaminodiphenyl sulfone	100 mg daily self-administered	
2. Clofazimine	300 mg once a month supervised and 50 mg daily self-administered	2 years or preferably, till smear negativity
3. Rifampicin	450–600 mg once a month, supervised	

fragmented *M. leprae*, a reminder of the underlying setting of ll leprosy. Subcutaneous histoid lesions display cytomorphological features identical to that of dermal lesions, differing only by their location. Following treatment, regressing lesions lack circumscription and resemble infiltrative lesions of ll leporsy, the cytoplasm of the macrophages becomes distinctly foamy. Acid-fast bacilli may not be demonstrable.

TREATMENT

Histoid leprosy patients should be treated on the same lines as per the recommendations of the WHO for multibacillary cases (Table 9.1).

RECOMMENDED READING

1. Anonymous. Expert Committee on Leprosy. Sixth Report. Technical Report Series No. 768. WHO. Geneva; 1988;14.
2. Sehgal VN, Srivastava G, Beohar PC. Histoid leprosy—a histopathoogical reappraisal. *Acta Leprol*. 1987;5:125-131.
3. Sehgal VN, Srivastava G, Saha K. Immunological status of histoid leprosy. *Lepr Rev*. 1985;56:27-33.
4. Sehgal VN, Srivastava G, Singh N. Histoid Leprosy: histopathological connotations relevance in contemporary context. *Am J Dermatopathol*. 2009;31:268-271.
5. Sehgal VN, Srivastava G. Histoid Leprosy. *Int J Dermatol*. 1985;24:286-292.
6. Sehgal VN, Srivastava G. Histoid leprosy. *Int J Dermatol*. 1985;24:286-292.
7. Sehgal VN, Srivastava G. Histoid Leprosy; a prospective diagnostic study in 38 patients. *Dermatologica*. 1988;177:212-217.
8. Sehgal VN, Srivastava G. Status of histoid leprosy-a clinical, bacteriological, histopathological and immunological appraisal. J Dermatol. 1987;14:38-42.
9. Sehgl VN, Srivastava G, Singh N, Prasad PV. Histoid leprosy: the impact of the entity on the postglobal leprosy elimination era. *Int J Dermatol*. 2009;48:603-610.
10. Singh N, Bhatia A, Tickoo SK, Arora VK, Gupta K. Negative-staining, refractile mycobacteria in Romanowsky-stained smears. *Acta Cytol*. 1994;39:1071.
11. Singh N, Bhatia A, Tickoo SK, Arora VK, Gupta K. Negative-staining, refractile mycobacteria in Romanowsky-stained smears. *Acta Cytol*. 1994;39:1071.
12. Wade HW. The Histoid variety of lepromatous leprosy. *Int J Lepr*. 1963;31:129-142.

10

Borderline (Dimorphous) Leprosy

Borderline (dimorphous) leprosy forms an important group in the evolution of leprosy. It includes borderline tuberculoid (BT); borderline borderline (BB) and borderline lepromatous (BL) of Ridley and Jopling's classification. Here the immunological behavior of the host shows fluctuations. Hence, it is an unstable group of leprosy. Its global prevalence is variable and approximates with that of lepromatous leprosy. It affects both males and females, and is commonly seen between 20 and 59 years of age.

CLINICAL FEATURES

It is a disease affecting the skin, nerves and also the systemic organs. The patients may report with the history of progressive changes in the color of the skin; tingling and numbness, crusting or recurrent bleeding from the nose, inability to appreciate hot and cold, and trophic changes such as blisters, ulcers, weakness, wasting and contractures. The wrist and footdrops may also be the presenting features.

Skin lesions: Examination of the skin surface in the broad daylight may reveal bizarre skin lesions resembling tuberculoid patches on the one hand, and macules or indurated lesions of lepromatous on the other. The lesions are a few to numerous. They are largely bilateral, but may be asymmetrical. The ill-defined as well as –defined lesions are the hallmark of the disease (Figs 10.1 to 10.5). Some of them may be erythematous shiny, while the others may be dry and scaly. A few of the lesions are smooth and are

markedly indurated with central hypopigmented or atrophy, characteristic of tuberculoid lesions. Other lesions may have induration with the usual soft and succulent features like that of lepromatous leprosy (Figs 10.6 to 10.32). They are widely distributed all over the body, but the ear lobes may be spared.

Sensations: The sensory disturbances may also present a bizarre pattern. Some of the lesions resembling tuberculoid may elicit hypoesthesia or anesthesia, especially marked at the center. Similar sensory changes may be seen in the peripheral part of the extremities.

Nerves: Cutaneous as well as the peripheral nerves are usually enlarged, but less frequently than tuberculoid. The trophic changes are seen only in

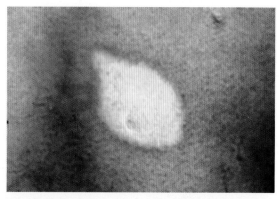

Fig. 10.1: Borderline tuberculoid: Hypopigmented, well-defined infiltrated patch with serrated margins located on the back. The sensations of temperature, touch and pain were impaired

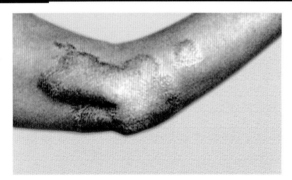

Fig. 10.2: Borderline tuberculoid: Hypopigmented, erythematous, well-defined lesion located near the elbow. Three satellite lesions were seen around it. The sensations of temperature, touch and pain were impaired. The nerve proximal to the patch was thickened and tender. The smear for AFB negative

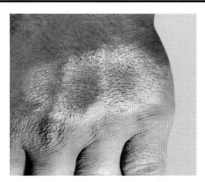

Fig. 10.5: Borderline tuberculoid: An erythematous indurated lesion with irregular margins and spares hair, located over the dorsum of the hand. Sensations were totally lost over the patch. Superficial nerve proximal to the lesion is thickened and tender, AFB negative

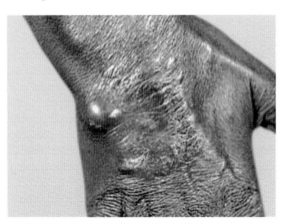

Fig. 10.3: Borderline tuberculoid with nerve abscess

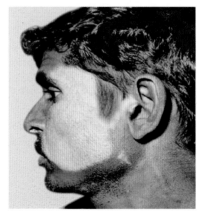

Fig. 10.6: Borderline tuberculoid: Located on the left cheek. Thickened greater auricular nerve of the same side, AFB negative

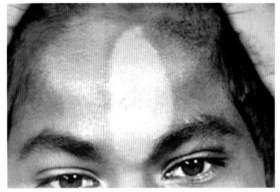

Fig. 10.4: Borderline tuberculoid: A hypopigmented patch with serrated margin located over the forehead. The patch is anesthetic. The left superaorbital nerve was thickened and tender, AFB negative

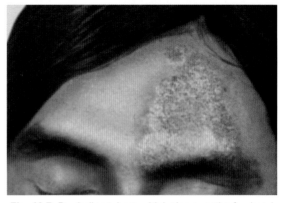

Fig. 10.7: Borderline tubercuoid: lesion over the forehead

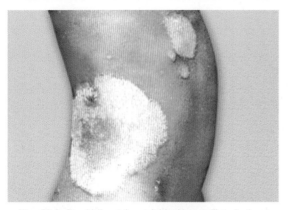

Fig. 10.8: Borderline tuberculoid with satelliete lesions

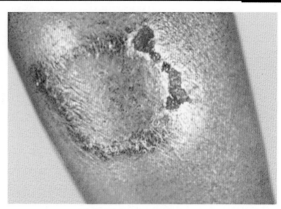

Fig. 10.11A: Borderline tuberculoid: An erythemato-scaly infilterated plaque with serrated borders and crusting at places over the forearm

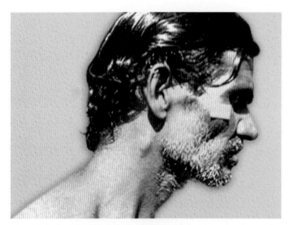

Fig. 10.9: Borderline tuberculoid: Lesions over the face with thickening and tenderness of left greater auricular nerve. A swelling along its course—nerve abscess

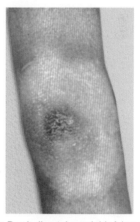

Fig. 10.11B: Borderline tuberculoid: A hypopigmented irregular patch having satellite lesions over the elbow

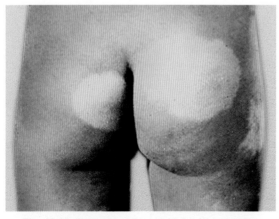

Fig. 10.10: Borderline tuberculoid: Lesions over the buttocks

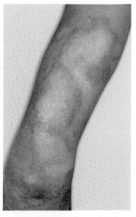

Fig. 10.11C: Borderline tuberculoid on the elbow

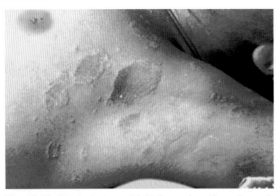

Fig. 10.12: Pityriasis rosea: Multiple, oval, erythemato-scaly lesions—the scaling being prominent at the periphery—along the body cleavages

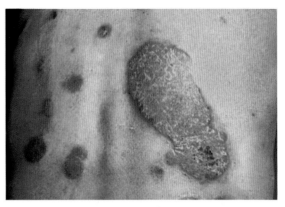

Fig. 10.15: Psoriasis: Well-defined erythemato-scaly, plaque, Auspitz sign positive

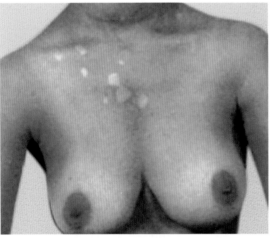

Fig. 10.13: Pityriasis varsicolor: Multiple hypopigmened mildly scaly macules of varying sizes present over the chest. Sensations are preserved. KOH preparation: positive

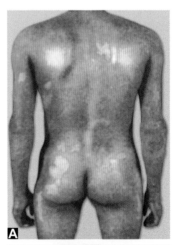

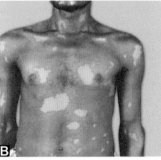

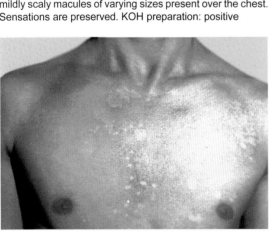

Fig. 10.14: Pityriasis versicolor

Figs 10.16A and B: Borderline borderline: Multiple, yet countable, hypopigmented, erythematous and scaly patches, some of them were well-defined and large, while the smaller lesions were merging imperceptible into the surrounding skin. The lesions were located on the back. Similar lesions were seen on the front of chest and abdomen. The sensations were either impaired or lost in these patches. The superficial nerves were thickened and tender, AFB Negative

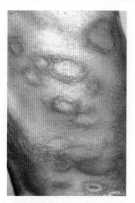

Fig. 10.17: Borderline borderline: Numerous, yet countable, erythematous, indurated, well-defined lesions with central depression (punched out lesions). A few lesions were indurated, erythematous and ill-defined. They were located on the trunk. In majority of lesions the sensory deficit was well-elicited, AFB negative

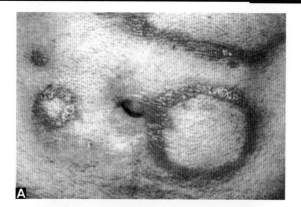

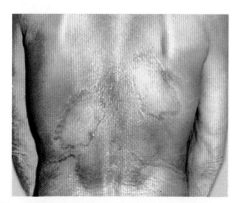

Fig. 10.18: Borderline borderline located on the back

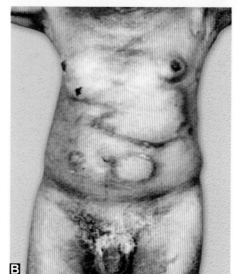

Figs 10.20A and B: Borderline borderline lesions on the trunk

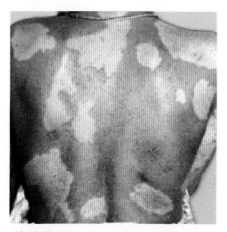

Fig. 10.19: Borderline borderline located on the back

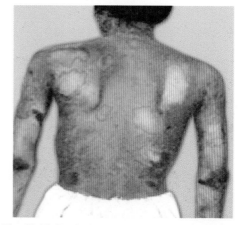

Fig. 10.21: Borderline borderline lesions on the back

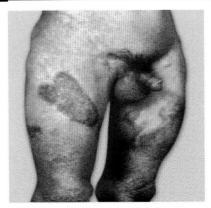

Fig. 10.22: Borderline borderline lesions on the trunk

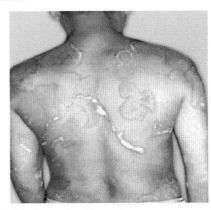

Fig. 10.25: Psoriasis: Well defined, erythemato-scaly lesions on the back: scaling marked at the periphery. Auspitz sign positive

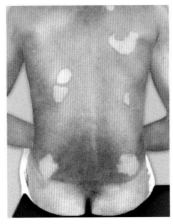

Fig. 10.23: Borderline borderline lesions on the back

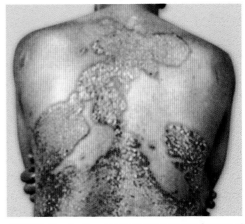

Fig. 10.26A: Psoriasis vulgaris lesions on the front or chest

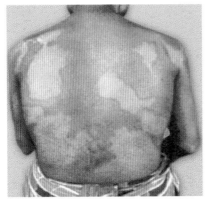

Fig. 10.24: Borderline borderline lesions over the back

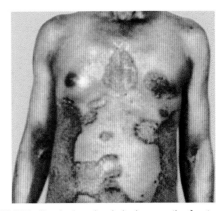

Fig. 10.26B: Psoriasis vulgaris lesions on the front or chest

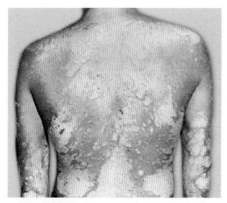

Fig. 10.27A: Psoriasis lesions on the back

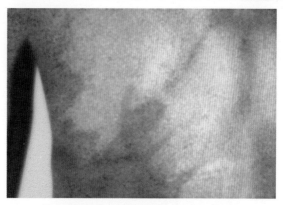

Fig. 10.29: Borderline lepromatous leprosy

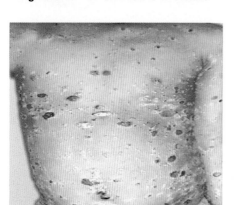

Fig. 10.27B: Psoriasis lesions on front of the chest

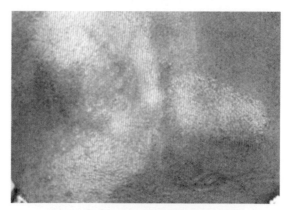

Fig. 10.30: Borderline lepromatous leprosy

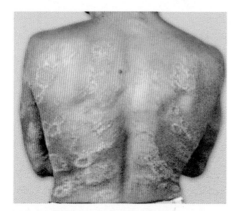

Fig. 10.28: Borderline lepromatous: Numerous, erythemato-scaly lesions of varying configuration—some conforming to tuberuloid morphology, while the large majority resembled lepromatous leprosy. Lesions were located over the back, almost bilaterally symmetrically. The sensations in the well-defined lesions were either impaired or lost, while in others there was no sensory deficit. The ulnar, radial and lateral popliteal nerves were thickened and/or tender

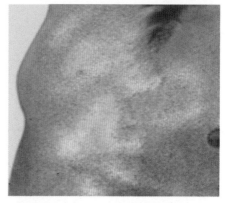

Fig. 10.31: Borderline lepromatous leprosy

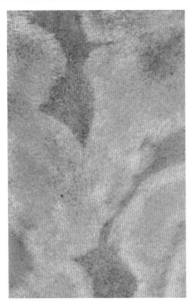

Fig 10.32: Borderline lepromatous leprosy

Table 10.1: Chemotherapy for multibacillary (MB) leprosy			
Clinical types	*Drugs*	*Dosage and mode of administration*	*Duration*
BT, BB, BL	Rifampicin	600 mg once monthly supervised	2 years or preferably till smear negativity
	Dapsone	100 mg daily self-administered	
	Clofazimine	300 mg supervised every month and 50 mg daily self administered	

advanced cases. They are described in 'neurotrophic manifestations of leprosy'.

Bacteriology: The routine-slit-skin smears may show moderate (+) to large number (+++) of lepra bacilli. However, the number of bacilli may vary in different lesions.

Lepromin test: It is variable and shows fluctuations.

Diagnosis

It is imperative to examine the patient carefully in broad daylight, lest the diagnosis may be overlooked. The presence of cardinal features of tuberculoid as well as lepromatous leprosy in the same patient or in the same lesions, helps in the diagnosis. The confirmation may, however, be done by the salient histological features as described in the preceding text.

Differential Diagnosis

While examination such lesions, the clinical features of tuberculoid and lepromatous type of leprosy should be reviewed. Their characteristic clinical features and diagnosis are discussed in the respective chapters.

▌TREATMENT

Borderline leprosy should be managed with multi-drug therapy according to its status. Borderline tuberculoid (BT), borderline borderline (BB) and borderline lepromatous (BL) cases should be treated as multi-bacillary leprosy. The details of regimen are shown in Table 10.1.

▌RECOMMENDED READING

1. Sehgal VN. Clinical criteria for the diagnosis of Hansen's disease. *The Star*. 1990;14:16.

Indeterminate Leprosy

Indeterminate leprosy group has been given due consideration in the different classifications of leprosy. It comprises early hypopigmented macule(s). They are poorly evolved, lacking the characteristics of well-determined lesions. In due course, they may develop into any of the well-recognized types of leprosy. These lesions, being early asymptomatic, may be missed or overlooked. They may occur in any age group, both in males and females, but their frequency is more amongst children.

CLINICAL FEATURES

Skin surface is largely affected.

Skin lesions: They are usually solitary, two or three hypopigmented, poorly defined macule(s), the margin being hazy, merging into apparently normal adjoining skin (Figs 11.1 to 11.3). The surface is usually uneven, but seldom dry and smooth (Table 11.1).

Sensations: The sensory disturbances may be equivocal.

Nerves: The regional nerves are apparently normal.

Bacteriology: Slit-skin smears are generally negative and may occasionally be positive.

Variants

The macules may show erythema. Hypopigmented and erythematous macules may be found in the same patient.

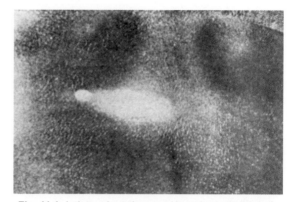

Fig. 11.1: Indeterminate leprosy: Hypopigmented macule over the back

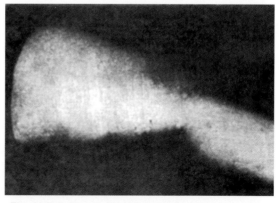

Fig. 11.2: Indeterminate leprosy: Hypopigmented bizarre macule on the thigh

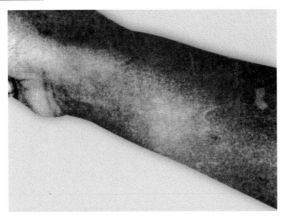

Fig. 11.3: Hypopigmented poorly defined macules (*Courtesy:* Sehgal VN, et al. *Int J Lep.* 1977;45:360)

Table 11.1: Clinical features	
Type	*Macule*
Color	Hypopigmented/ erythematous
Margins	Vague and ill-defined
Infiltration	Absent
Surface	Not dry, may be smooth
Sensations	Equivocal
Temperature	Impaired, with exceptions
Light touch	Frequently not impaired
Pain	Impaired, with exceptions
Nerve thickening	Usually, absent rarely +
Number	One, few or a few
Location	Buttocks, thighs, trunk, extensors

Diagnosis

It is difficult clinically. Histopathology, however, may be of assistance.

Differential Diagnosis

While suspecting indeterminate group, it is worthwhile to recapitulate the characteristic clinical presentation of maculo-anesthetic leprosy and macules of lepromatous leprosy. Other skin conditions such as pityriasis simplex, pityriasis versicolor, previtiligo and post-inflammatory hypopigmentation should form

its differential diagnosis. The salient clinical features of these conditions are described below.

Pityriasis simplex: It is clinically recognized as ill-defined, hypopigmented, asymptomatic macules usually located on the face, amongst children. The condition is transitory, and occurs in malnourished persons. It is a subliminal infection of the skin due to *Staphylococcus albus*. The absence of the cardinal clinical features of leprosy helps in its exclusion.

Pityriasis versicolor: It is characterized by asymptomatic hypopigmented, mildly scaly, multiple macules distributed on the body surface, corresponding largely to the 'lady's bathing suit' Seasonal variation is its feature. The diagnosis is confirmed by finding mycelia and spores of *Malassezia furfur* when the scrapings are seen under the microscope.

Previtiligo: It is the initial stage of vitiligo wherein there is an insidious loss of pigmentation of the skin. The lesions are hypopigmented and ill-defined. They may progress to form ivory white macules—classical of vitiligo. There is no loss of hair or sweating or disturbance of sensations. Thickening and/or tenderness of the regional nerves is lacking.

Post-inflammatory hypopigmentation: The lesions are hypopigmented with ill-defined margins. They are the remnants of various inflammatory dermatoses. The history of inflammatory dermatoses is affirmative. The history of inflammatory dermatoses is affirmative and of course, characteristic clinical features of leprosy are lacking.

▌TREATMENT

Once the diagnosis of indeterminate leprosy has been made with absolute confidence, all cases should be treated by administering 1–2 mg/kg body weight/day of dapsone in unsupervised daily doses, and 10 mg/kg body weight/day of rifampicin monthly supervised for a period of 6 months. After the regimen the treatment may be stopped. The patient should then be kept under regular surveillance for a period of 3 years. However, it is imperative to monitor the results of this treatment with great care.

▌RECOMMENDED READING

1. Arnold HL Jr. How indeterminate leprosy got its name? *Int J Dermatol*. 1981;20:393-395.
2. Bechelli LM. Indeterminate leprosy in a population survey and in the subsequent follow-up of children. Congress Abstract Paper XII. *Int J Lepr*. 1984;52:685.
3. Brownie SG. Self healing leprosy: report of 2749 patients. *Lepr Rev*. 1974;45:104-111.
4. Fajardo TT. Indeterminate leprosy—a 3-year study, clinical observations. *Int J Lepr*. 1971;39:94-95.
5. Fajardo TT. Indeterminate leprosy—a five study, clinical observations. Abstract of Congress papers 18/156. *Int J Lepr*. 1973;41:576.
6. Sehgal VN, Srivastava G. Indeterminate leprosy. A passing phase in the evolution of leprosy. *Lepr Rev*. 1987;58:291-299.
7. Sehgal VN. Clinical criteria for diagnosis of Hansen's disease. *The Star*. 1990;14:16.

12 Polyneuritic Leprosy

Polyneuritic leprosy is an accepted entity, which manifests itself by neural signs without any clinical evidence of skin lesions. It corresponds to pure neuritic varieties of *Madrid Classification*. The immunological behavior in this type may be variable. It occurs all over the world, and this entity is well-recognized in the Indian subcontinent. It affects both males and females, of all age groups.

CLINICAL FEATURES

It may manifest either as primary polyneuritic or secondary polyneuritic leprosy. In primary polyneuritic, many peripheral nerves are affected, without any evidence of present or past involvement of the skin. Secondary polyneuritic leprosy, on the other hand, is associated with quiescent scars of old skin lesions. Similar affection of a single nerve is described as primary or secondary mononeuritic leprosy.

Invariably the patient reports with the complaints of progressively increasing numbness and tingling, sensation of pins and needles, heaviness and inability to appreciate sensations. Radiating pains may also be the presenting feature. Aforesaid symptoms usually start from the peripheral parts of the extremities, extending upwards in the later course of the disease. Recurrent blistering of the hands and feet with formation of ulcers may frequently be present. Weakness, wasting and contractures may also be reported in advanced cases.

Peripheral nerves: the peripheral nerve(s) are enlarged. The extent of involvement may vary. The whole nerve trunk may be thickened or it may be localized. The localized enlargement of the nerve is likely to form a nerve abscess(s) (Figs 12.1 to 12.5). It is chronic, and show, it takes a long

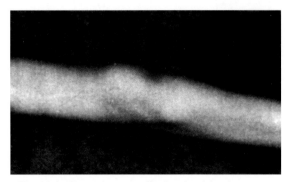

Fig. 12.1: Nerve abscess, affecting the right ulner nerve

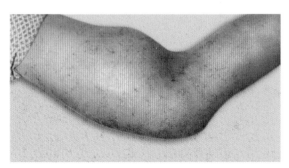

Fig. 12.2: Nerve abscess of the right ulner nerve

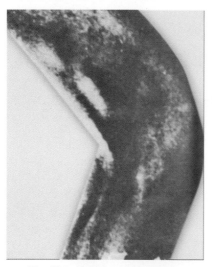

Fig. 12.3: Multiple nerve abscess

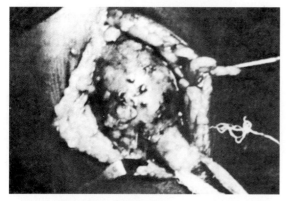

Fig. 12.4: An exposed nerve abscess
(*Courtesy:* Sehgal VN Leprosy Review, 1966;37:109)

time to develop. It represents essentially a good immunological response on the part of the host against *Mycobacterium leprae* trying to limit the disease process. Subsequent trophic changes in the muscles supplied by the affected nerve, is in direct proportion to the muscles to the pressure caused by the abscess on the nerve fibres. At times, however, the nerve abscess shows spontaneous healing or opens on the skin, a rare situation. The tenderness of the nerves is a cardinal feature. One or more nerves may be affected, but the common nerves involved are the ulnar, radial, median in the upper extremities, while lateral popliteal, and posterior tibial in the lower. In addition, greater auricular

(Figs 12.6A to C), fifth and seventh cranial nerves may also get involved.

Sensations: The disturbance of the sensory modalities is a cardinal sign, and it depends upon the extent of involvement of the nerves. Impairment or loss of sensation usually occurs along the disturbance is vital, temperature sensation is affected first, followed by touch and pain. The deep sensations are last to be affected. Furthermore, asymmetrical sensory disturbance is an important sign in neuropathy due to leprosy. Glove and stocking type of anesthesia may be present.

Motor changes: They are noticed as weakness, wasting, atrophy and contractures of the muscles. The site of affliction depends upon the nerve involved. The affliction of the ulnar nerve produces anesthesia in its distribution, paresis and wasting of the small muscles of the hand, causing flattening of hypothenar eminences, and guttering of interosseous spaces. Further, it may produce various deformities-difficulties in adduction of little finger, difficulty in flexion of the little and ring finger at the metacarpophalangeal joints—a typical claw hand. The affliction of the median nerve may produce anesthesia of the lateral half of the palm,

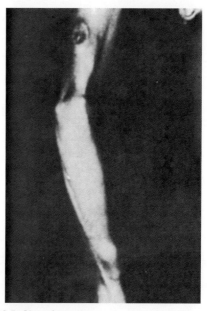

Fig. 12.5: Sinus formation on the nerve abscess—a rare situation

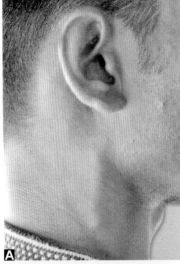

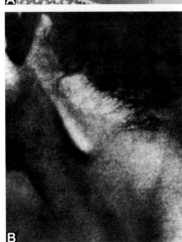

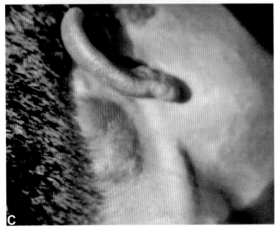

Figs 12.6A to C: Thickening of the greater auricular nerve

wasting of the thenar eminence and paralysis of the muscles supplied by the median nerve below the wrists. There is clawing of all the fingers, and inability of the thumb to abduct or oppose the fingers in grasp or pitch when both the nerves are involved. Similarly, affliction of the radial nerve may cause wrist drop.

Various deformities of the foot are produced when the lateral popliteal nerve is affected. Hypoesthesia or anesthesia of the dorsum of the foot and the outer side of the leg and paresis of the peroneal and the extensor muscles may lead to footdrop. High stepping gait is cardinal. The involvement of posterior tibial nerve produces anesthesia of the sole of the foot, keratosis and trophic ulcers. Repeated trauma, pressure, and secondary infection further worsen the situation causing destruction, both of soft and bony parts. The details of clinical manifestations are described in 'neurotrophic manifestations of leprosy'.

The afflictions of the fifth and seventh cranial nerves are described under 'ocular leprosy'.

Reflexes: The deep reflexes are either normal or exaggerated. They are seldom lost, in striking contrast to peripheral neuropathy due to other causes.

Diagnosis

It is based on the cardinal features of thickening and/or tenderness, and absence of skin lesions. Hypoesthesia or anesthesia in the distribution of the affected nerve is contributory. The confirmation of the diagnosis may be done by the histological pattern seen in the nerve.

Differential Diagnosis

Many a times other conditions may create a problem in the diagnosis of poly-or mono-neuritic leprosy. Consideration of salient clinical features of peripheral neuritis, maralgia paresthetica, hypertrophic interstitial neuritis and primary amyloidosis of the nerves may be important conditions in the differential diagnosis.

Peripheral neuritis: History of diabetes mellitus, excessive and prolonged consumption of alcohol, and ingestion of drugs containing heavy metals, is helpful. In addition, there is bilateral symmetrical glove and stocking type of anesthesia, tenderness of calf muscles and nerves (without enlargement), and diminution or loss of deep reflexes. The clinical features of polyneuritic leprosy are, however, wanting.

Meralgia paresthetica: It is localized neuritis of the lateral cutaneous nerves of the thighs. It is characterized by paresthesia/anesthesia without any apparent skin change along the distribution of the nerve, on the outer aspect of the upper thigh. It is a self-limiting condition. It lacks the classical clinical features of leprosy.

Hypertrophic interstitial neuritis: It is rare familial sensory neuropathy characterized by thickened, hard, and tender peripheral nerves. Progressive trophic manifestations indistinguishable from those caused by leprosy are associated features. The histological examination of the affected nerve is imperative to exclude, and differentiate it from leprosy.

Primary amyloidosis of the nerves: It is a rare congenital progressive disease of the peripheral nerves. It is characterized by the absence of cutaneous sensibility; the peripheral nerves are normal in size and are non-tender on palpation. Histopathology of nerves is of immense value in its diagnosis.

TREATMENT

The treatment of primary polyneuritic leprosy is in no way different from that of pauci-or multibacillary leprosy. However, the status of the disease should be clearly established. In view of the occurrence of motor and sensory damage causing drastic complications, it is worthwhile to be careful in treating these patients.

The duration of therapy is variable, and depends upon the clinical response, and the activity of the disease, characterized by gradual diminution of tenderness and thickening of the nerve. It may be desirable to continue the treatment for a period of two to three years after the control of the activity.

In addition to specific treatment, surgical intervention may be needed to relieve nerve pain and to prevent irreversible damage. Decompression of the thickened nerves in the unyielding bony or facial canals, when undertaken in early stages, may be helpful. Simple division of compression bands is advocated. In a completely paralyzed nerve, however, epineurectomy is justifiable to relieve intractable pain.

RECOMMENDED READING

1. Sehgal VN. Clinical criteria for the diagnosis of Hansen's disease. *The star*. 1990;14:16.

13

Leprosy in Children

Leprosy in children forms an important link in the study of natural evolution of the disease. Infants and young children in families of infective leprosy patients are considered "high risk group". In such individuals, therefore, a single or a few exposures to infective parents may be sufficient to transmit the infection. Further, children are more susceptible for the immune system is not fully developed. The children are more susceptible for the immune system is not fully developed. The children of low socioeconomic status are its frequent victims. Incubation period is variable. The age at onset of the disease is usually between 5 and 14 years. Leprosy in children is equally prevalent in both the sexes.

▌ CLINICAL FEATURES

Leprosy may manifest in one of the four ways, namely, cutaneous lesions, neural symptoms, reactional episodes and deformities/trophic changes. In children, reactional episodes and deformities/trophic changes are seldom presenting features. The patient usually reports with asymptomatic or hypoesthetic skin lesions, and less commonly with neural manifestations. Although the onset of leprosy is insidious, yet it is interesting that sometimes the appearance of early lesions in borderline (dimorphous) leprosy may be ushered in by general malaise and slight pyrexia. However, these prodromal symptoms are rarely identifiable and have no clinical or diagnostic significance. Hypopigmented macules, infiltrated raised plaques,

lichenoid papules, papulonodules and weal-like papules may be recorded in that sequence.

Indeterminate leprosy: It is recognized by a bizarre hypopigmented, dry, mildly scaly, faintly erythematous macule. Sweat response and hair usually remain unaffected. Margins in indeterminate leprosy are either ill-or well-defined. There may or may not be a sensory deficit (Fig. 13.1). The nerves supplying of feeding the patch are apparently spared. Usually a single macule is its feature. Occasionally several asymmetrically disposed macules may also be seen. The lesions are usually present on the buttocks, trunk and proximal parts of the extremities. Due to their trivial and

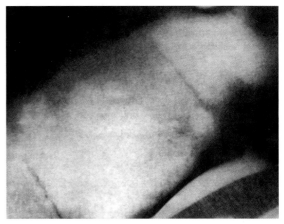

Fig. 13.1: Indeterminate leprosy: Hypopigmented macule with irregular margins

asymptomatic nature, the macules of indeterminate leprosy are frequently overlooked.

Tuberculoid leprosy: It is another well-established clinical form of the disease in children. It usually expresses itself in the form of macule(s). The macules are either hypopigmented or erythematous. Occasionally, they may show pigmentation in the center. The marines of the lesions are either clearly defined or irregular. The macules are dry, scaly and anhidrotic. Sensations of temperature, touch and pain are either impaired or completely lost. The regional nerves supplying to, or feeding the patch are enlarged and/ or tender, a finding in contrast to that of indeterminate leprosy. A raised, erythematous, uniformity/partially indurated plaque, with demarcated regular borders and completely absent or impaired sensations, may occasionally be seen in children.

Borderline leprosy: Borderline tuberculoid (BT) leprosy is frequently encountered. However, mid-borderline (BB) and borderline lepromatous (BL) are observed only occasionally. The lesions of borderline leprosy found in children largely correspond to those seen in adults, but they are primarily constituted by macular (Figs 13.2 to 13.4) rather than infiltrated plaques. Although the impairment of sensations may be found in BT, yet it may be absent in BB lesions.

Lepromatous leprosy: This entity is sparingly seen in children. More often than not, an occasional case of indeterminate leprosy may directly land into lepromatous leprosy in children with clinical features as described earlier.

Neuritic leprosy: The salient neurological symptoms are enlargement of the superficial nerve trunks, with or without pain and tenderness and loss of sensations in areas supplied by them.

Sites of affliction: The sites for the development of the first lesion of leprosy in children appears to be peculiar, and are localized primarily on the buttocks or thighs, followed by arms, forearms, legs and lumbar region.

Reactional episodes: These are unusual and hence the information on the subject is incomplete and does not clearly delineate their clinical features. However, in such a situation the criteria for their diagnosis shall be the same as for adults.

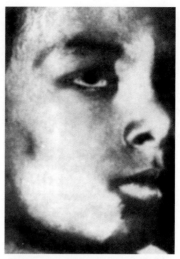

Fig. 13.2

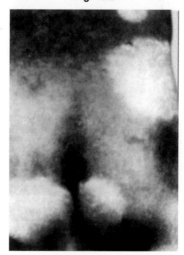

Fig. 13.3

Figs 13.2 and 13.3: Borderline leprosy: Hypopigmented mildly scaly macule

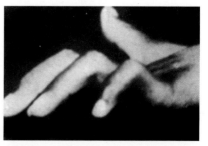

Fig. 13.4: Claw hand in borderline leprosy

Course of the disease: The course of untreated leprosy in children is largely unpredictable. A see-saw battle between the immunological responses and the organism is lucidly reflected by the waxing and waning character of the lesions. One type of lesion may transform into the other. Indeterminate leprosy, a frequently encountered clinical manifestation amongst children, may remain unchanged, heal spontaneously or progress to evolve itself into any of the determinate groups/types of leprosy. Thus, a strict surveillance is indicated in every case of childhood leprosy.

Diagnosis

At the very outset, it may be emphasized that the diagnosis of leprosy in children should only be made when the symptoms and signs of the disease are unequivocal. It is imperative to consider clinical, bacteriological, histopathological and immunological features while diagnosing leprosy.

The clinical features of leprosy may sometimes be confusing in children. A further difficulty may arise, while eliciting the sensory, sweat and hair loss over the patch in infants and very young children. However, the sensation can be tested in children as young as 3–4 years provided their confidence is gained, and they understand what we want to know. Similarly, impairment of sweating may be ascertained if the child is exposed to the sun (heat) for a while which may induce sweating. Slit-skin smears and nasal swabs seldom yield a positive result in children. Nonetheless, they should always be performed, at least in suspected multi-bacillary child. Slit-skin smears are usually negative in over 90 percent of the affected children, infiltrated lesions may, however, be positive for *M. leprae*. Similarly, histopathology may sometimes be unrewarding in early tuberculoid or indeterminate leprosy. Furthermore, a disparity between the clinical and the histopathological features may be explicit. Macular lesions in particular are usually offset with

this disparity. Nevertheless, histopathology forms a vital tool in classifying a nondescript lesion. Special staining procedures may reveal a few acid-fast bacilli along a small nerve twig or in the vicinity of skin adnexae despite slit-skin smear negativity.

In every child, lepromin test (early Fernandez and late Mitsuda)—should always be performed. It is positive in 20 percent children under 5 years, and 60 percent up to 10–14 years of age. Further, its negativity in children with positive fluorescent leprosy antibody absorption (FLA-Abs) test, heralds the chances of development of a multi-bacillary leprosy. A proportion of these children may be classified as "at risk" when FLA-Abs test is positive, with a doubtful or negative lepromin. Their frequency may serve as an index of susceptibility to leprosy in certain population.

Serum radioimmunoassay (SRIA) has recently been utilized for demonstration and quantitation of anti-mycobacterial antibodies in the cord sera of children of mothers with leprosy. This technique can be utilized in defining the population "at risk" and for following the progression of prodromal stages of leprosy into manifest disease or its resolution.

▌TREATMENT

The treatment of leprosy in children is similar to that of adults. However, the drug dosage has to be regulated according to the body weight. Multi-drug therapy (MDT) forms its basis (see Table 13.1). The opinion regarding the administration of treatment in indeterminate leprosy where lepromin (Mitsuda reaction) is negative, and FLA-Abs test is complementary. It is necessary to emphasize that indeterminate leprosy with strongly positive lepromin may be followed inquisitively to establish its natural evolution. However, treatment in the latter is not indicated. Furthermore, the emergence of resistant strains of *M. leprae* should be borne in mind for which periodic clinical and laboratory assessment is necessary.

Table 13.1: Multidrug therapies (MDT) of leprosy in children

Drugs	Dosage	Frequency	Supervision	Duration
Paucibacillary Diaminodiphenyl sulfone Rifampicin	1–2 mg/kg/day 10 mg/kg/day	Daily Once monthly	Self-administered Supervised	6 months 6 months
Multibacillary Diaminodiphenyl sulfone	1–2 mg/kg/day	Daily	Self-administered	24 months or till smear negativity
Rifampicin	10 mg/kg/day	Once monthly	Supervised	
Clofazimine	1–2 mg/kg/day	Monthly loading dose* and daily dose	Supervised Self-administered	
Indeterminate				

FLA-Abs +ve: Lepromin +ve No treatment required.

FLA-Abs –ve: Lepromine –ve: treat as multi-bacillary leprosy.

*In adults, the monthly loading dose 300 mg and the daily dose is 50 mg.

RECOMMENDED READING

1. Noussittoo FM, Snsrric H, Wlter J. Leprosy in children. World Health Organization, 1st edn, Geneva: 1976.
2. Sehgal VN, Joginder, Jain VK, Prakash SK. Cell-mediated and humoral immunity in leprosy in children. *J Dermatol* (Tokyo). 1990;17:356-361.
3. Sehgal VN, Joginder. Leprosy in children, correlation of clinical, histopathological, bacteriological and immunological parameters. *Lepr Rev*. 1989;60:202-205.
4. Sehgal VN, Rege VL, Mascrenhs MF, Reys M. The prevalence and pattern of leprosy in a school survey. *Int J Lepr other mycobact Dic*. 1977;45:360-363.
5. Sehgal VN, Sehgal S. Leprosy in young urban children. *Int J Dermatol*. 1988;27:112-114.
6. Sehgal VN, Srivastava G. Leprosy in children. *Int J Dermatol*. 1987;26:557-566.

14

Reactions in Leprosy

Leprosy, a chronic infective granulomatous condition, presumptively caused by *Mycobacterium leprae*, usually runs an uneventful course. At times, the course of the disease may be punctuated by exacerbation of the existing lesions and/or appearance of new lesions. This has now been designated as reaction in leprosy. With the advances in immunology, reactions have become a focus of attention. Also, there has been a controversy regarding its terminology. The reactions at the present juncture should be classified into type I (lepra) and type II (erythema nodosum leprosum). The former is delineated into type I upgrading/ reversal and downgrading reaction. This reaction embraces unstable components comprising BT, BB, and BL of the continuous leprosy spectrum. TT and LL are usually spared. Type II (ENL) occurs in BL and LL groups of leprosy. Occasionally BB may also be affected (Figs 14.1A and B).

▮ MECHANISM

Type I (lepra) reaction: The immunologically unstable, borderline group, (BT, BB, BL) exhibit type I (lepra) reaction. The immunologically stable polar groups (TT and LL), however, do not show this reaction. Acute shifts incell-mediated lymphocytic immunity precipitate type I reaction. It is an expression of delayed hypersensitivity, and represents type IV (Cell-mediated) hypersensitivity

reaction of Gell and Coomb. It occurs as a result of interaction of T-lymphocytes with antigens liberated from disintegrating *Mycobacterium leprae*. It may be triggered by various precipitating factors such as:

1. MDT comprising dapsone, rifampicin, clofazimine
2. Drugs like Vitamin A, iodides, bromides
3. Intercurrent infection like streptococcal, malaria, filarial and other causes of pyrexia
4. Tetanus, BCG and other vaccinations.
5. Pregnancy, puerperium and lactation.
6. Physical, physiological and psychological stress.

The presence of competent T-lymphocytes is mandatory for development of type reaction.

During type I (upgrading/reversal) reaction, an augmented *in vitro* lymphocyte response to

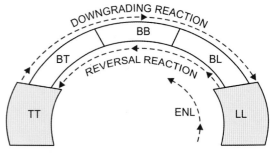

Fig. 14.1A: Mechanism of reaction in leprosy

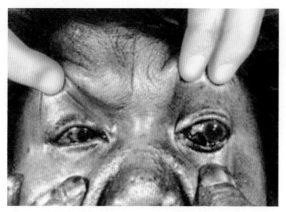

Fig. 14.1B: Erythema nodosum leprosum reaction showing iridocyclitis

Type I (Downgrading) reaction

Type I (Downgrading) reaction
1. Loosening of the granuloma
2. Granuloma pushed down in the dermis
3. Relatively free subepidermal zone
4. Increasing macrophages in granuloma, moderate epitheliod cells and lymphocytes
5. Giant cells conspicuously absent
6. Increase in AFB
7. Edema of collagen fibers manifested as progressive lightening of eosinophilic staining of dermis

M. leprae antigens is recorded through lymphocyte transformation test (LTT) and lymphocyte migration inhibition test (LMIT), reflecting an increase in cell-mediated immunity. Also, the lepromin test becomes strongly positive, while the bacillary index (BI) may fall. There is a significant increase in T lymphocytes, which returns to normal after the reaction subsides. In BT and BB patients, the most likely time for upgrading reaction to occur is during 6 months after starting treatment. If the reaction is associated with a reduction of CMI, it is considered as downgrading reaction. The resultant imbalance between the hypersensitivity and bacterial load is responsible for the manifestation of downgrading reaction. The type I reaction is a mirror image of ameliorating or deteriorating CMI in borderline group.

Histopathology

Type I (upgrading) reaction
1. Well-formed compact granuloma
2. Granuloma approximates the epidermis
3. Exocytosis
4. Free sub epidermal zone tends to be obliterated
5. Increase in epitheliod cells and lymphocytes
6. Occasional or a few giant cells
7. Reduction in AFB
8. Edema of collagen fibres manifested as progressive lightening of eosinophilic staining dermis

Type II (ENL) reaction: Increased host response to the bacilli is its primary cause. However, it may be precipitated by antileprosy drugs namely dapsone, clofazimine, and rifampicin. The organisms and their breakdown products combine with the antibodies to form complexes, which activate complement which in turn liberates the mediators of inflammation. Potassium iodide, vitamin A and progesterone may also cause this phenomenon. Immunological suppression during puerpureum, small-pox, and tetanus and BCG vaccination may also precipitate the reaction. Inter-current infections such as streptococcal, malaria, filarial, and intestinal infestation may provoke the reactional state. They may also be precipitated by physiological and psychological stress.

Type II (ENL) reaction
1. Dilatation of upper dermal blood vessels
2. Perivascular neutrophilic infiltration of lower dermal and subcutaneous vessels
3. Extravasation of RBC
4. Dermal edema
5. Scanty, granular AFB
6. Endothelial cell proliferation and obliteration of the lumen, prominent in erythema nodosum necroticans

Clinical features: The clinical diagnosis of type I (lepra) reactions, therefore, should be clearly understood and formed around the clinical criteria which are characterized by:
1. Erythema
2. Edema, 'inverted saucer' instead of the saucer the right way up

3. Hyperalgesia
4. Expansion of the existing lesions
5. Ulceration
6. Excruciatingly tender and thickened regional nerves.

In case, one or a couple of lesions show the preceding changes with or without ulceration, it is recognized as an upgrading (reversal) reaction (Figs 14.2 to 14.5). Paresis and/or paralysis of the muscles supplied by the affected nerves may be apprehended in the upgrading reaction. While these changes affecting almost all lesions, it is designated, as type I (downgrade) reaction (Figs 14.6 to 14.8). In addition, appearance of fresh lesions may also be associated with constitutional symptoms such as pyrexia, malaise, loss of appetite and joint pain. At this juncture it is imperative to differentiate type I (downgrading) reaction from downgrading *per se* (Table 14.1), a situation envisaged in the continuous leprosy spectrum, largely affecting the borderline group.

Type II (ENL) reaction is diagnosed on the basis of sudden appearance of erythematous, tender, evanescent cutaneous and/or subcutaneous nodules. Occasionally, the nodules may ulcerate to form erythema nodosum necroticans. The lesions are usually distributed over the extensors of the body. Remissions and exacerbations are their hallmark.

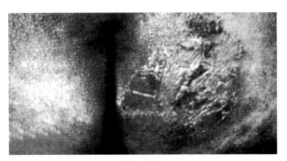

Fig 14.2

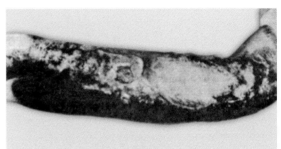

Fig 14.3

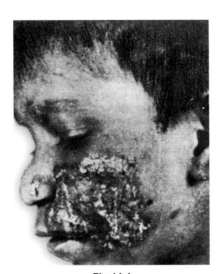

Fig 14.4

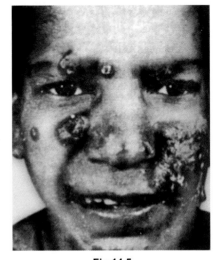

Fig 14.5

Figs 14.2 to 14.5: Type I (upgrading) edema, desquamation and ulceration of the lesion

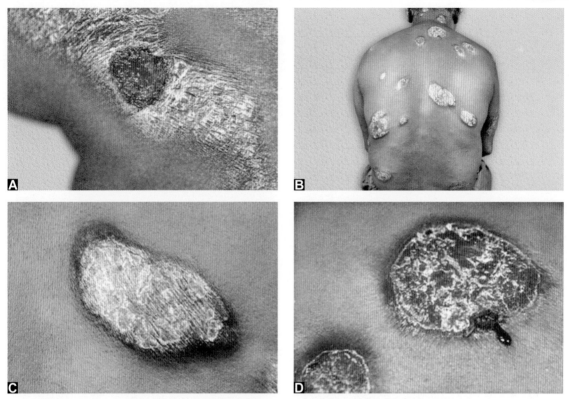

Figs 14.6A to D: Borderline lepromatous: Numerous, indurated, scaly, raised lesions of varying sizes, some of them showing erosions located on the back, depicting downgrading reaction

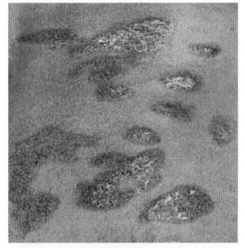

Fig. 14.7: Borderline lepromatous leprosy in downgrading reaction

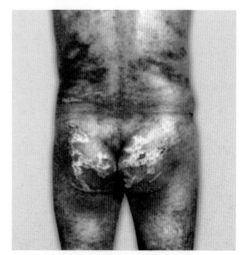

Fig. 14.8: Borderline lepromatous leprosy showing downgrading reaction

Table 14.1: Criteria for downgrading reaction and downgrading *per se**

	Downgrading reaction	*Downgrading per se*
Morphology	• Lesion in downgrading reaction show	• Change in morphology as follows
	– Erythema	– From well-defined to ill-defined
	– Edema	– Irregular or serrated margins
	– "Inverted saucer" appearance	– New satellite lesions
	– Expansion of lesions	• Conspicuous absence of edema and tenderness
	– Appearance of new lesions	
Number	Increase in number of lesions	Increase in number of lesions beyond 3 to uncountable
Nerves	Excruciatingly tender enlarged nerves	Increase in number of nerves involved, may or may not be tender
Bacterial Index	BI may or may not show significant changes	BI increases from 0–2 to 4–5
Lepromin	May of may not change significantly	Lepromin changes from +++ to –
Histopathology	Granuloma shows Loosening of granuloma Increase in histiocytes Absence if giant cells Decreases in lymphocytes Granuloma pushed down to mid or lower dermis Edema of collagen fibres manifested as progressive lightening of eosinophilic staining of dermis	Granuloma shows similar changes as in downgrading reaction; however, edema is conspicuously absent

*(Sehgal *et al.* relapse or later reversal reaction. *Int J Lep*, 1990;58:118–120.

Peripheral nerves when affected become tender and enlarged (Figs 14.9 to 14.13). Systemic involvement in the form of conjunctivitis, keratitis, iritis, iridocyclitis, hepatosplenomegaly, orchitis and enlargement of lymph nodes should be looked for as its manifestation. Marked constitutional, symptoms characterized by fever, malaise, anorexia, arthralgia and myalgia may be the distressing features.

LUCIO Phenomenon: It is an intriguing manifestation of erythema nodosum leprosum reaction usually seen in untreated or relapsing lepromatous patients. It is characterized by an extensive, bizarre, painful ulceration of the skin usually unaccompanied by constitutional symptoms. It largely occurs in pure, primitive, diffuse lepromatosis (PPDL) often referred to as spotted leprosy of Lucino. This is primarily seen in Costa Rica and the Sinaloa and Jallisco provinces of Mexico. The onset of the Lucio phenomenon is a gradually spreading purplish erythema, which then forms a hemorrhagic infarct or plaque followed

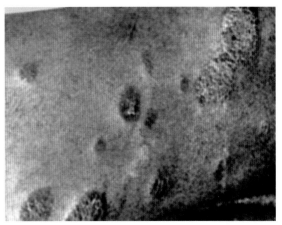

Fig. 14.9: Borderline lepromatous leprosy in downgrading reaction

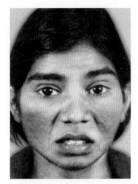

Fig. 14.10: Erythema nodosum lesions on face

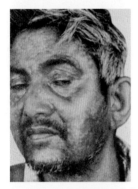

Fig. 14.11: Erythema nodosum leprosum lesions on face

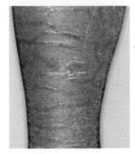

Fig. 14.12: Icthyosis over the legs in a patient with erythema nodosum leprosum

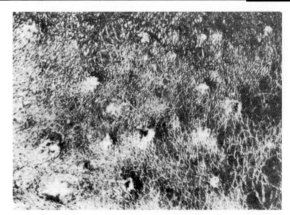

Fig. 14.13: Type II (ENL) numerous nodules of varying sizes, some of which are showing necrosis

TREATMENT

It differs in type I (Lepra) and type II (ENL) reactions. However, it may be conceived that multidrug therapy must be continued according to paucibacillary/multibacillary status of the disease.

Type I (Lepra) Reaction

Upgrading (reversal): Usually 40–60 mg of prednisolone daily in two divided doses, at 9 am in the morning and 6 pm in the evening, is administered. The improvement in the condition is assessed by regression in clinical signs of activity namely decrease in erythema and/or edema in the lesion, decrease in the tenderness and/or thickening of the affected nerve. The duration of the treatment may vary from 2–4 weeks. Clofazimine (Hansepran, Lamprene) may be a useful anti-inflammatory adjuvant to the preceding therapy. It should be administered in the dosage of 200–300 mg daily. It not only supplements in action of prednisolone, but also helps in tapering of its dose by its steroid-sparing action.

In case, a nerve in a fibrous canal is affected, it is likely that the response to the above treatment may not be prompt. In that eventuality, neurolysis should be considered.

Down grading: It should be treated in a similar fashion as that of reversal reaction. Constitutional symptoms should preferably be managed by administering requisite dosage of aspirin. Chloroquine

by a blister. The blister ruptures to form a bizarre ulcer with 'jagged' margins. Such lesions occur extensively over the legs, thighs, forearms and buttocks. The ravages of the disease are evident as atrophic scars. Constitutional symptoms are conspicuously absent. Bacterial endotoxins, stress and strains may exacerbate or precipitate the condition. Recurrences during winter are common. Systemic amyloidosis may be a terminal event.

diphosphate may be useful in mild cases. It is available in 250 mg tablet containing 150 mg of the active ingredient. A three weeks schedule consisting of three tablets per day for first week, two tablets per day for second week and one tablet per day for the third week is adequate.

Type II (ENL) Reaction

Glucocorticoids (prednisolone) form the main stay for its management. 60–80 mg of prednisolone in two equally divided doses, morning 9 am and evening 6 pm, is administered for a variable period. This is supplemented by an augmented dose of clofazimine which may range from 200–300 mg per day. The favorable response to the treatment is recorded by regression of existing lesions and absence of fresh lesions. This usually takes 4–6 weeks following which prednisolone is tapered step-wise, 5 mg every third or fourth day. The patient may be maintained from 15–20 mg of prednisolone per day along with 100 mg of clofazimine. Maintenance therapy is successful in preventing the recurrences of ENL. In case the response to oral prednisolone is not prompt, parenteral dexamethasone (Decadron) may be a handy alternative. One ml (4 mg) may be injected intramuscularly or intravenously morning and evening for a similar duration.

Thalidomide, if available, is useful in controlling ENL. 100–200 mg daily at bed time is generally adequate. In case it fails in the above dosage, prednisolone and/or clofazimine may be needed in addition. Its teratogenecity drastically restricts its use. Sleepiness, visual disturbances and peripheral neuropathy are its other side effects. The drug is absolutely contraindicated in females of child bearing age.

Lucio phenomenon requires intensive supportive care as well as vigorous antibacterial and anti-inflammatory therapy. Plasmapheresis may be needed when other means are ineffective.

▌RECOMMENDED READING

1. Bjune G. Reactions in leprosy. *Lepr Rev.* 1983;61-67.
2. Ramu G, Ramanathan VD. Reactions in Hansen's disease—A reappraisal. *The Star*, 1990;49:7-11.
3. Rea TH. An overview of reactional status in Hansen's disease (HD). *The Star*, 1989;48:1-5, 13.
4. Sehgal VN, Gautam RK, Koranne RV, Beohar PC. The histopathology of type I (lepra) and type II (ENL) reactions in leprosy. *Indian J Lepr.* 1986;58:240-243.
5. Sehgal VN, Sharma V. Reactions in leprosy--a prospective study of clinical, bacteriological, immunological and histopathological parameters in thirty-five Indians. *J Dermatol* (Tokyo). 1988;15:412-419.
6. Sehgal VN, Srivastava G, Sharma VK. Contemplative immune mechanisms of Lucio phenomenon and its global status. *J Dermatol* (Tokyo). 1987;14:580-585.
7. Sehgal VN, Srivastava G, Sundharam JA. Immunology of reactions in leprosy. Current status. *Int J Dermatol.* 1988;27:157-162.
8. Sehgal VN. Clinical criteria for diagnosis of reaction in Hansen's disease. *The Star*, 1990;50:14-15.
9. Sehgal VN. Reactions in leprosy. Clinical aspects. *Int J Dermatol.* 1987;26:278-285.
10. Waters MF. Turk JL, Wemambu SN. Mechanism of reactions in leprosy. *Int J Lepr Other Mycobact Dis.* 1971;39:417-428.

15

Ocular Leprosy

Ocular involvement is a frequent manifestation of leprosy. *Mycobacterium leprae* may either affect the eye directly or indirectly. The direct involvement occurs in lepromatous and borderline leprosy, while indirect is seen in tuberculoid and polyneuritic leprosy. The latter is due to the affliction of the fifth and seventh cranial nerves.

It is observed all over the world, but the pattern of ocular changes may vary in different endemic belts of the world. Almost 25 percent of the leprosy patients may have one or other manifestations of the disease. The eye may be implicated in both sexes, at all ages though predominantly in the older age group. The duration of the disease seems to play a significant role in ocular involvement. Longer the duration of leprosy, more are the chances of the eye manifestations.

CLINICAL FEATURES

They depend upon the mode of infection-direct or indirect nevertheless the presenting complaints may be similar. The patient may report with loss of eyebrows or eyelashes, irritation, lacrimation, redness, inability to close the eye, white spots, diminishing vision and blindness.

When the ocular changes are secondary to involvement of fifth and seventh cranial nerves the following eye changes may be seen.

Indirect Secondary Involvement

Trigeminal nerve: In case the trigeminal nerve is affected, there is loss of sensation of conjunctiva and cornea, which may lead to loss of the protective mechanism of the eye. This may cause exposure conjunctivitis and keratitis with the attending symptoms.

Facial nerve: The infiltration of the facial nerve may cause infra-nuclear type of paralysis. It is characterized by lagophthalmos due to paralysis of the orbicularis oculi and ectropion of the lower lid (Fig. 15.1), which predisposes to exposure keratitis. Side by side the muscles of the lower part of the face may be affected producing signs, namely, dribbling of saliva, flattening of nasolabial folds, inability to whistle, drawing up of the angle of the mouth to the opposite side and absence of wrinkling of the forehead (Figs 15.2 to 15.4).

The signs of conjunctivitis, keratitis and corneal ulcers may be seen (Fig. 15.5). Secondary infection

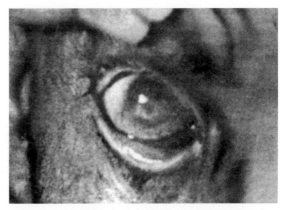

Fig. 15.1: Lagophthalmos, ectropion and corneal opacity

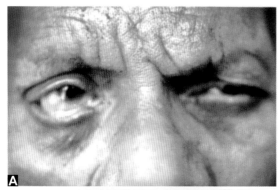

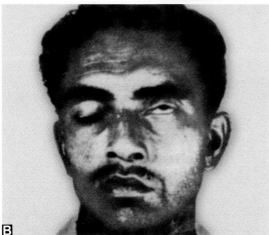

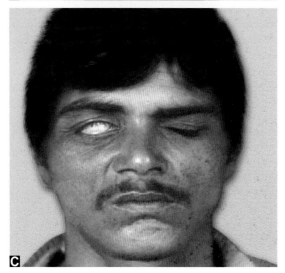

Figs 15.2A to C

of the latter may cause iritis, iridocyclitis or even panophthalmitis.

A simultaneous involvement of trigeminal and facial nerve may be complementary in furthering the eye damage (Figs 15.6 to 15.10).

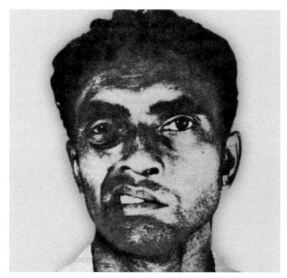

Fig. 15.3

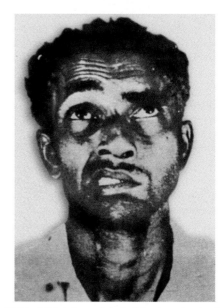

Figs 15.2 to 15.4: Infranuclear facial palsy, showing lagophthalmos, deviation of the angle of the mouth and loss of wrinkles on the forehead

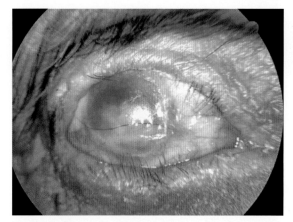

Fig. 15.5: Exposure keratitis, corneal opacity and ectropion

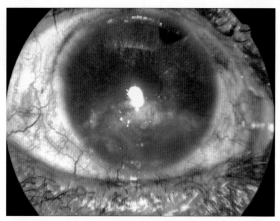

Fig. 15.8: Occular leprosy: Legophthalmos and exposure keratitis

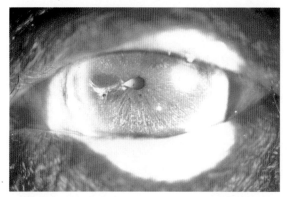

Fig. 15.6: Ocular leprosy: Atrophic iris scar/distortion of pupil

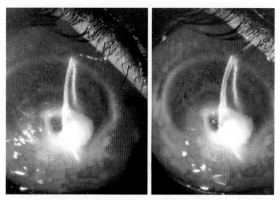

Fig. 15.9 Ocular leprosy: Corneal perforatin with synechia at perforated site

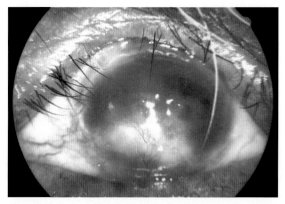

Fig. 15.7: Ocular leprosy: Vascularized corneal scar, upper lid distortion and trichiasis

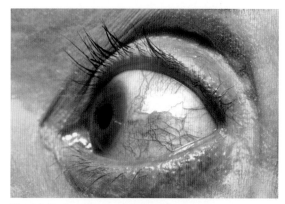

Fig. 15.10: Ocullar leprosy: Ectropian with chronic conjunctivitis

Direct Eye Involvement

The tissues of the eye may be affected by the direct spread of *Mycobacterium leprae* through the blood stream and/or extension of the skin lesions. The salient clinical features of involvement of different parts of the eye are described below:

Eyebrows: The hypertrophy and the loss of hair from the lateral one-third of the eyebrows is a cardinal feature. These manifestations are due to induration of the skin and infiltration of the hair follicles. Similarly, eyelashes may be affected.

Eyelids: Formation of nodules and hypertrophy of the eyelids is common, giving them a smooth and shiny appearance. Massive infiltration of the eyelids may cause difficulty in opening eyes.

Conjunctiva: A mild, chronic conjunctivitis is often seen with the presenting symptoms of photophobia, irritation, lacrimation and redness. Examination of the eye may reveal congestion and at times nodules of varying sizes on the conjunctiva. They are smooth reddish and non-tender. The involvement of deep subconjunctival tissue may result in episcleral nodules, a cardinal sign of eye involvement.

Cornea: It is frequently affected. Initially it may be asymptomatic, but in the later course of the disease, severe disturbance of vision may be complained of. Beaded appearance of the nerves in the cornea is the earliest sign, followed in due course by superficial punctuate keratitis (SPK), pathognomonic of leprosy. It is characterized by localized, discrete, milky, chalky deposits on the cornea. Pannus formation is common. It extends around the entire corneal circumference—a feature peculiar to leprosy. Eventually, it may lead to a sclerosing keratitis, extending, and right around the limbus. Perforation of the cornea is uncommon until secondary bacterial or viral infection supervenes.

Sclera: This is usually affected as a part accompaniment of superficial punctuates keratitis, iritis and iridocyclitis. It is seldom affected alone.

Iris and ciliary body: They are commonly affected and may manifest in the form of military lepromatous—'iris pearls', nodular lepromata, chronic plastic iridocyclitis, and acute diffuse plastic iridocyclitis. One or combination of all the preceding lesions may be seen in the same patient.

Miliary lepromata: They are tiny, white spots in the iris formed by aggregations of lepra bacilli. They are found immediately adjoining the papillary margin. They are pathognomonic, and also assist in the early diagnosis of ocular leprosy.

Nodular lepromata: They are multiple, yellowish nodules of varying sizes, seen over the iris. They occur infrequently.

Chronic plastic iridocyclitis: This is the most frequent involvement of leprosy. Its insidious onset and chronicity are its hallmark. Clinical examination of the eyes may reveal keratotic precipitates on the back of the cornea, and exudates in the anterior chamber and on the anterior lens capsules. There may be an occlusion of the pupil. It is small and irregular, non-reacting to light or accommodation. The latter is due to formation of multiple posterior synechiae. Later, cataract, vitreous opacities, retinal detachment and atrophy of the eyeball—phthisis bulbi—may be seen. Glaucoma is, however, unusual; such changes are responsible for progressive diminution of vision and eventual blindness.

Acute diffuse plastic iridocyclitis: This may be precipitated by dapsone therapy as a part accompaniment of erythema nodosum leprosum. Its onset is acute and associated with pain, watering, redness, photophobia and failing vision. Circumcorneal congestion and a non-reacting, small fixed pupil are its diagnostic clinical signs.

Posterior segment: Until recently, the involvement of posterior segment of the eye was unknown. Recently, it has been described to affect the choroids and retina in the form of white, waxy, refractile deposits and also lesions similar to those of iris pearls' But, occurrence of such lesions is extremely uncommon.

Diagnosis

The diagnosis of ocular lesions of leprosy depends upon their morphological characteristics. The nature of these lesions—direct or indirect/secondary—is, however, determined by the type of leprosy. Furthermore, the demonstration of lepra bacilli from the lacrimal fluid and/or conjunctival scraping is supplementary. The emphasis must be given to the early ocular manifestations of leprosy in order to prevent severe disturbance of vision and eventual blindness.

TREATMENT

It is imperative to establish the bacteriologic (pauci- or multibacillary) status in each case. Accordingly, multidrug therapy should be instituted. Management of extra ocular and ocular lesions preferably should be done under the care of an expert ophthalmologist. Madarosis and blepharochalasis require plastic repair, in which an island neurovascular pedicle graft is used in the former and a plastic repair and brow lift is done in the latter. Entropion and ectropion should be surgically corrected.

As soon as lagophthalmos is detected, a course of systemic corticosteroids (30–40 mg prednisolone) should be administered to recover the nerve function. The cornea and conjunctiva at this stage should be effectively protected from exposure and dryness. Lubricating drops such as methyl cellulose 2 percent, sterile liquid paraffin, or castor oil should be administered to the eyes frequently, as should a bland eye ointment. The bland eye ointment should be applied to the eyes before going to sleep. In outdoor activities, care should be taken against injuries, bright light and exposure. A bandage should never be applied, because it may further damage the insensitive cornea. Should there be no perceptible recovery of lagophthalmos by the preceding measures, a surgical intervention may be imperative. If the corneal sensations are maintained, a temporalis muscle transfer or tarsorrhaphy "(using tarsorrhaphy lid clamp) should be performed. If the corneal sensations are impaired, then a mechanical closure of the eyelids is indicated.

Corneal ulceration should be managed by conventional antibodies and mydriatics. With the advent of recent topical mydriatics such as tropicamide cyclopentolate and phenylephrine, however, the situation seems to have changed. A temporary stitch on the eyelids or tarsorrhaphy is an essential adjuvant to provide adequate rest to the damaged cornea. Use of topical corticosteroids in corneal ulcer should be scrupulously avoided. Visual improvement achieved by repositioning of pupil in corneal morbidity by a noninvasive technique (using low energy argon laser photocoagulation of mid/peripheral iris) is promising in the achievement of relief from corneal disability.

Iridocyclitis should be managed vigorously to avoid permanent damage to the vision. A topical mydriatic should be administered twice daily to provide requisite rest and to prevent the formation of posterior synechia. Systemic corticosteroids, 30–40 mg of prednisolone, should be given along with topical application of steroids.

RECOMMENDED READING

1. Ffyrche TJ. Role of changes as a cause of blindness in lepromatous leprosy. *Br J Ophthalmol.* 1981;65:231-239.
2. Lamba PA, Kumar DS. Ocular involvement for leprosy. *Indian J Ophthalmol.* 1984;32:61-63.
3. Lamba Pa, Srinivasan R, Rohtagi J. Surgical Management of ocular leprosy. *Ind J Ophthalmol.* 1987;35:153-157.
4. Sehgal VN, Lamba PA. Ocular changes in leprosy. *Int J Dermatol.* 1990;29:175-182.
5. Shield Ja, Warring GO 3rd Monto LG. Ocular findings in leprosy. *AM J Ophthalmol.* 1974;77:880-890.

16

Deformities and Disabilities in Leprosy

Leprosy has been regarded as a dreaded disease manifesting as gross disabilities, deformities and mutilations. Even at present great human suffering and a substantial loss of manpower results from the development of deformities in an overwhelming number of leprosy patients. This aspect has attracted the attention of several investigators all over the globe. WHO defines impairment as the abnormality or loss of psychological, physiological or anatomical structure or function; disability is the restriction or lack (resulting from impairment) of ability to perform an activity in a normal manner or within the range considered normal. Disability has also been defines as a deterioration of one's ability or capacity to perform a function normally. Deformity, on the other hand, is an alteration in the form, shape or appearance of the affected part of the body.

Deformities have been classified according to the five-grade classification of the World Health Organization (WHO) which provides clear-cut delineation. This classification, therefore, needs to be followed in such studies in institution, whereas the recently introduced three-grade classification may be a boon for paramedical workers in the field. This may provide fresh incentive to organize and evolve uniform research pattern so that effective corrective measures could ultimately be devised.

GRADING OF DEFORMITIES/ DISABILITIES

The WHO classification of deformities/disabilities forms a convenient tool for their grading. The deformities/disabilities of the hands, feet and face should preferably be evaluated separately. It is worthwhile at this juncture to recall briefly the applied anatomy of the hands and feet.

Nerve Supply of the Hands

Sensory nerve supply: The sensory nerve supply of the hands is through the ulnar and the median nerves. The former supplies medial 1.5 fingers while the latter supplies the remaining 2.5 fingers and the thumb.

Motor nerve supply: The median nerve supplies the various muscles in the forearm and hand. These are the pronator teres, flexor carpi radialis, palmaris longus, flexor digitorum superficialis, flexor policies longus, lateral half of flexor digitorum profoundest, and pronator quadrates in the forearm, and abductor pollicis brevis, flexor pollicis brevis, opponens pollicis and the first and second lumbricals in the hand. The ulnar nerve deals with the movements. After supplying a part of flexor digitorum profundus in the forearm, it gives branches to the short muscles of the hand (palmaris brevis, abductor digiti minimi, opponens and flexor digiti minimi, 3rd and 4th lumbricals four each of palmar and dorsal interossei and two parts of abductor pollicis).

NERVE SUPPLY OF THE FEET

Sensory nerve supply: The dorsum of the foot is supplied by the superficial peroneal nerve which distributes its branches to all the toes except the adjacent side of the first and second toe, which is supplied by the deep peroneal nerve, and the lateral side 5th toe which is supplied by the sural nerve. In the sole, the medial plantar nerve supplies 3.5 digits on the hallux side, whereas the lateral plantar nerve supplies the remaining digits. The skin under the heel is supplied by the medial calcaneal branch of the posterior tibial nerve.

Motor nerve supply: The medial plantar nerve supplies the abductor hallucis, flexor digitorum brevis, flexor hallucis brevis and the lumbricals in the sole, while the rest of the muscles including 7 interossei and abductor hallucis are supplied by the lateral popliteal nerve supply tibialis anterior, extensor digitorum longus, extensor hallucis and peroneus tertius. The medial popliteal nerve, on the other hand, supplies plantaris, medial and lateral heads of gastronemius, soleus and popliteus.

GRADING OF HAND DEFORMITIES

Grade I: For defining this deformity, the sensation of temperature, touch and pain should be meticulously tested. Should they be absent, it is classified as grade I deformity.

Grade II: Claw hand with functional thumb indicates Grade II deformity (Figs 16.1 to 16.4). This should be confirmed by testing various muscles of the hand. Care must be taken to choose only

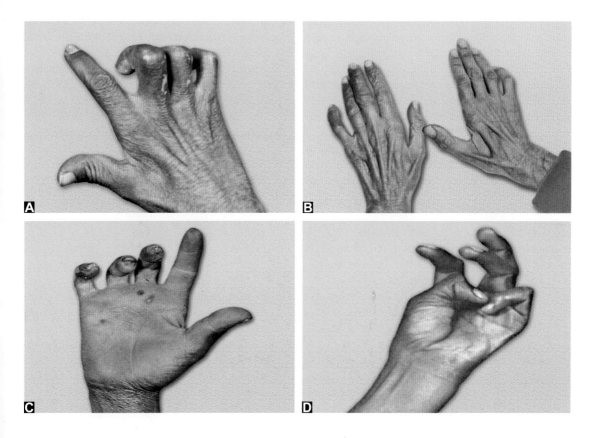

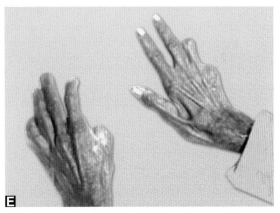

Figs 16.1A to E: Flattering of the hypothenar eminences and guttering of ntersseous spaces (Grade II deformity)

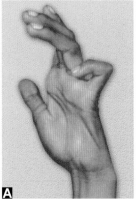
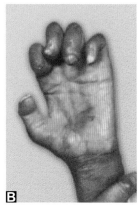

Figs 16.3A to B: Flattering of the hypothenar eminence of the hands (Grade II deformity)

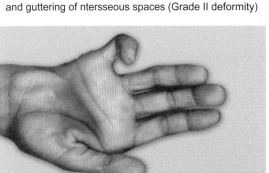

Fig. 16.2: Mobile claw hand: useful thumb (Grade II deformity)

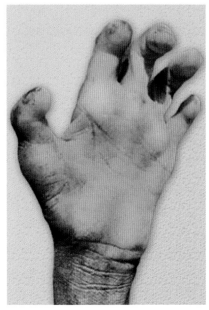

Fig. 16.4: Clawing of the finger with fixed thumb (Grade III deformity)

those movements which are either guarded by a single muscle or a number of muscles supplied by the same nerve. Muscles supplied by the median nerve are:

a. *Abductor pollicis brevis:* It is tested by asking the patient to place the dorsum of the hand on the table with palm facing upwards. He is asked to touch the pen held in front of the thumb. Inability to touch it indicates paralysis.

b. *Opponens pollicis:* The patient is asked to touch the tip of his thumb across the palm. The absence of this movement indicates loss of motor function of this muscle.

c. *Flexor pollicis longus:* The patient is asked to bend the terminal phalanx of the thumb, while the proximal phalanx is held firmly to eliminate the action of short flexors. Inability to flex the terminal phalanx indicates paralysis of this muscle.

Muscles supplied by the ulnar nerve are:

a. *Palmar and dorsal interossei:* The patient is asked to abduct and adduct the fingers. Further, he is asked to straighten the 2nd and 3rd phalanx after steadying the first phalanx. If the preceding movements are absent, it indicates their paralysis.

b. *First palmar interosseous and abductor pollicis:* The patient is asked to hold a book between the thumb and fingers. Flexion of terminal phalanx is indicative of their paralysis (Froments' sign).

Grade III: It is characterized by the paralysis of the intrinsic muscles resulting in contractures (Fig. 16.5). This is tested by passively flexing the fingers. Less than 25 percent of passive range of movements confirms the presence of contractures.

Grade IV: It is identified by the partial absorption of the fingers but their useful length is retained (Fig. 16.6).

Grade V: Gross absorption of the fingers with only small stumps as their relics, denotes Grade V deformity (Fig. 16.7).

GRADING OF FOOT DEFORMITIES

Grade I: Loss of sensation of temperature. Touch and pain denotes this deformity of the foot.

Grade II: This is assigned in the event of present/past trophic ulceration of the foot (Figs 16.8 to 16.10)

Grade III: The functions of the medial and lateral popliteal nerves are tested in order to define this deformity.

Medial popliteal nerve: Its involvement is demonstrated by asking the patient to walk on the floor, watching carefully whether the heel first touches the floor, and also for any indication of loss of springing action. Further, the patient is asked to flex them, it indicates paralysis of muscles supplied by this nerve.

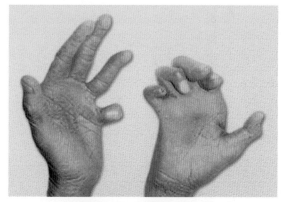

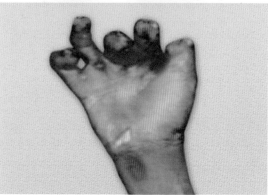

Figs 16.6 and 16.7: Mutilation of the hand (Grade V deformity)

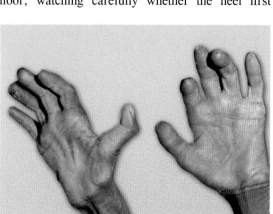

Fig. 16.5: Tropic ulcer of terminal phalanges of the hand causing resorption of the finger (Grade IV deformity)

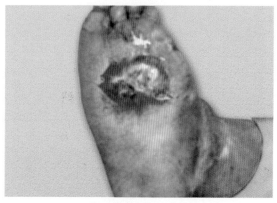

Fig. 16.8: Tropic ulcer

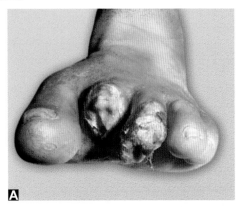

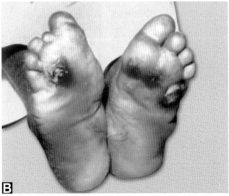

Figs 16.9A and B: Tropic ulcer over the head of metatarsal bones (Grade II deformity)

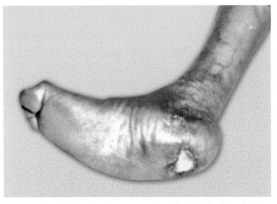

Fig. 16.10: Tropic ulcer occupying the heal of the foot (Grade II deformity)

Lateral popliteal nerve: These are tested by asking the patient to dorsiflex and evert the foot against resistance. Involvement of this nerve is indicates by inability to demonstrate these movements.

Grade IV: An absorption of the foot of less than 1/3 of the surface area of the sole points to grade IV deformity.

Grade V: When more than 1/3 of the foot is lost, it indicates grade V deformity.

GRADING OF FACIAL DEFORMITIES

Grade I: The presence of supraciliary madarosis, distortion or destruction of the cartilage of the ears or both, is classified as grade I deformity.

Grade II: It is assigned to patients with depression of the bridge of the nose.

Grade III: The loss of function of the VII cranial nerve serves as its indicator, which may be evaluated as follows:

The patient is asked to shut his eyes lightly. In cases of paralysis of the 7th nerve either the eyelids do not close as completely as on the less affected or unaffected side, or the eyes will deviate upwards to make up for the failure of the lids to close (Bell's phenomenon).

Patient is asked to whistle. In cases of paralysis, he is unable to do so.

He is asked to show his teeth. In paralysis of this nerve, the mouth is drawn toward the healthy side.

Grade IV: Loss of vision in one eye or dimness of vision in both eyes denotes grade IV deformity. Visual acuity is tested as per recommendations of the WHO.

A split circle, C, of 9 mm diameter and 2 mm thickness is drown in black ink on cardboard. Only one eye at a time is tested. A normal eye can see the gap in the circle from 6 meters distance. If the patient fails to appreciate this, the chart is brought progressively nearer to the eye, still, if he is unable to read it, then he is asked to count fingers. In the extreme cases, when this also is not possible, light is projected on the eye from different directions and he is asked to tell its direction. Failure to recognize even this means blindness of that eye.

Grade V: It is indicated by complete blindness of both eyes.

Other Deformities

Lepromatous leprosy patients should also be examined for laryngeal involvement by indirect laryngoscopy. Larynx, hypopharynx and epiglottis should be examined for dull-gray nodular infiltrations, ulceration, scarring contractures or both.

Epidemiology

Prevalence and incidence: The prevalence and incidence of deformities and disabilities vary from place to place in different studies. This is primarily due to varied prevalence rates of leprosy in general in different geographical areas. Nearly 25 percent of leprosy patients have some or the other form of disability.

Age: There has been a gradual lowering in the afflicted age group. Further, in younger patients, deformities primarily result either in TT or BT, as the same groups are common in younger people.

Sex: The frequent occurrence of deformities in men is partly due to their more afflictions with leprosy in general and partly on their indulgence in more manual work.

Occupation: Deformities and disabilities are usually found to be greater among manual workers, both unskilled and skilled. Evidently, they are more frequently exposed to repeated trauma and infections.

Education: The illiterate and the semiliterate are more prone to deformities and disabilities. This appears primarily due to ignorance about the disease, and lack of knowledge about the precautions required preventing deformities.

Socioeconomic standard: People of low socioeconomic strata predominantly suffer from deformities.

Type of disease: Generally, deformities are more common is lepromatous. This is primarily due to its diffuse nature, long silent course, involving most of the nerve trunks, with resultant fibrosis and damage on healing.

Duration of the disease: Deformities/disabilities usually occur when the patient has the disease for a relatively long period of time. The frequency of occurrence of deformities in all leprosy groups is directly proportional to its duration. However, deformities are shown to develop earlier in tuberculoid and borderline tuberculoid but fairly late in mid-borderline, borderline lepromatous and lepromatous leprosy. A longer duration of the disease evidently exposes the subject more to detrimental environment in addition to the infliction of more damage by the progressive disease itself.

Deformities of the hand: The hand forms the most common site of deformity in leprosy. Specific deformities include frozen hand, intrinsic plus finger and twisted fingers. They are chiefly seen in lepromatous leprosy. Motor paralytic deformities include claw fingers (intrinsic minus finger), adducted thumbs and dripped wrist and digits. They are chiefly seen in non-lapromatous patients, and after reactional episodes. Anesthetic deformities include scar contractures, stiffness and shortening of fingers, multination of hands, and disorganization of the wrist.

Deformities of the foot: They are the second most common deformities seen in leprosy. Specific deformities are fairly rare and comprise of reaction foot, twisted toes and intrinsic paralysis of toes. Motor paralytic deformities result from the paralysis of the intrinsic and extrinsic muscles of the foot, and include claw toes and footdrop. Anesthetic deformities include neuropathic planter ulceration and disorganization of the foot.

Deformities of the face: The most disfiguring deformity of the face, the nasal bridge depression, is seen primarily in lepromatous (LL) leprosy. Loss of eyebrows is seen only in lepromatous leprosy.

Development of gynecomastia: It is exclusively seen in lepromatous leprosy.

Laryngeal involvement: Laryngeal involvement primarily occurs in lepromatous leprosy.

▌PATHOGENESIS

Leprosy *per se* may not be responsible for most of the deformities/disabilities attributed to it. It precludes the sensation of pain, and thus encourages the patient to damage and deform himself. Recurrent trauma and subsequent secondary bacterial infections are the major offenders for the gross mutilations. Deformities have been classified into primary and secondary. Primary damage is directly due to the activity of the disease and the ensuing tissue response to the presence of *M. leprae.*

It is thus called specific deformity. The secondary damage is either inflicted by the patient himself or results from anesthesia, paralysis or other primary damage. Often, both the primary and secondary factors contribute to the deformity.

PRIMARY DEFORMITY

A widespread dissemination of acid-fast bacilli occurs throughout the body in lepromatous leprosy. In some tissues, their presence may not cause any damage, but in others considerable damage may result.

Nerve: Leprosy is primarily regarded as a disease of the nerves which are most susceptible to *M. leprae*. The bacilli may be identified in all peripheral nerve trunks, and occasionally in the dorsal root ganglia. However, there is no interference with the function of the central nervous system and the spinal cord. Damage to the peripheral nerves may result in motor and sensory loss. However, the pattern of nerve damage throughout the body is uniform. There may be perceptible damage to the motor function of the different nerves, namely the ulnar nerve just above the elbow or wrist, common peroneal nerve just above the neck of the fibula, posterior tibial nerve 3–4 inches above the ankle joint, zygomatic branch of the bony facial canal. Occasionally, the radial nerve may also be afflicted at the point of its emergence from under the triceps muscle. The nerves to the muscles of the shoulders, hips, trunk, neck and upper arm seem to be relatively immune to paralysis in leprosy.

Loss of sensation in leprosy is a major handicap due to its largely irreversible nature. It results both from the nerve trunk paralysis, and glove and stocking anesthesia caused by the involvement of cutaneous nerves. Anesthesia can also be demonstrated in skin lesions due to the involvement of the intracutaneous nerves. Bacilli have been demonstrated in all parts of the nerve fibers. Vater-pacini and Meissner sensory corpuscles may also be invaded by the acid-fast bacilli and later get atrophied and obliterated.

In every healthy skin, a constant process of nerve degeneration and regeneration continues. It is regularly seen in growing children, and in areas subject to repeated friction or preceding trauma. *M leprae* has a special predilection for the degenerating and regenerating nerve fibers. After their invasion, there occurs an accumulation of histiocytes around them, with invasion and fragmentation of the nerve fibers. Eventually, it leads to pigmentary, sensory and related local changes in the skin.

In cases of recent paralysis, the nerves get swollen due to edema and cellular infiltration. The type of infiltrate differs with the type of leprosy, as does the distribution of infiltrate between the epi-peri- and endoneurium. Swelling results in a relative ischemia of the nerve. Partial ischemia causes a reversible loss of conductivity of the nerves without Wallerian degeneration. The nerve is, however, destroyed if this partial ischemia lasts for long hours or, if there is a total ischemia. A stage of conduction block always precedes a true nerve function disturbance in leprosy. This may last upto a year, and may be followed by recovery. A reversible block can be distinguished from an irreversible one only through electrical tests. The most constant factor is the primary affliction of those nerves which are near the skin surface, without an overlying cover of a muscle, and thus having a temperature several degrees below the body core temperature. The factors predisposing to peripheral nerve involvement are: (i) superficial situation, (ii) overlying a bone, (iii) lying proximal to a rigid osteofacial canal and (iv) those subjected to alternate angular and stretch strains. Small nerve bundles containing only a few axons, although liable to infiltration and edema, yet seem to be less prone to paralysis. The difference between affliction of a thin and that of a thick nerve probably is that the amount of swelling surrounding a single nerve fibre is less likely to cause pressure than the same degree of swelling around each of a hundred or more nerve fibers all bound together in one sheath. In brief, the chief factors governing the paralysis of the infected nerve are: (a) the relationship of a patients' tissue with the type of disease. At one end of this scale is the lepromin-positive tuberculoid case highly susceptible to paralysis, while at the other is the lepromin-negative lepromatous case least prone to such damage. Thus, deformity always appears late in lepromatous leprosy; (b) the number of nerve fibers enclosed within the epineurium of the nerve. Numerous nerve fibres within the bundle augment the chances of paralysis; (c) the greater the perpendicular distance from the surface of the body, the lesser are the chances of paralysis.

Skin: Redundant and wrinkled facial skin is frequently seen in long-standing lepromatous laprosy. The skin of certain regions has a predilection to get more infiltrated. These are the face, ear lobules, forehead, eyelids, and maxillary and nasolabial areas. The infiltration results in gradual changes in the collagen and elastic fibers which ordinarily give shape and elasticity to the skin. They gradually disappear causing sagging of the skin. A distortion or destruction of the hair follicles may also take place.

Bones and cartilages: Bone changes have been documented in leprosy *M. leprae* may induce cystic bone changes. Bone cysts result from the destruction of bone trabeculae by the lepromas. Active formation of lepromatous granulation tissue and subsequent carious absorption and necrosis may be responsible for specific bone lesions of leprosy. A high concentration of lysosomal enzymes and acid-phosphatases has been demonstrated in patients with resorptive bone changes. Osteoclasts are incriminated in the extra-cellular release of acid phosphatases during bone resorption.

Facies leprosa, comprising atrophy of the anterior nasal spine alone or combined with atrophy of the central maxillary process was advanced by Mollar Christensen *et al.* Inflammatory changes of the superior surface of the hard palate may be an additional finding as is the affliction of cartilage of the nose. Lepromatous infiltration of the nasal mucosa is responsible for its ulceration leaving cartilage and bony framework to the environment. Secondary infection further hastens the process of exposure necrosis of the cartilage and bone, with eventual perforation and collapse of the nasal bridge.

Radiological bone changes have been documented time and again and aptly divided into specific and nonspecific changes, and osteoporosis. Specific bone changes of leprosy result from direct damage due to *M. leprae.* They have been broadly divided into two groups.

a. Lepra reactive group change varying from the terminal tuft dissolution to severe bone

destruction with resultant healing with bone sclerosis and twisted fingers. Occasionally, sub-periosteal bone erosion due to lepra reaction may be observed (Figs 16.11 to 16.15)

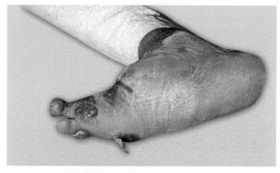

Fig. 16.11: Foot deformity. Grade IV

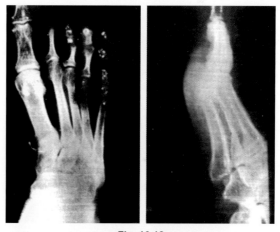

Fig. 16.12

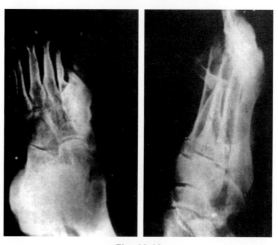

Fig. 16.13

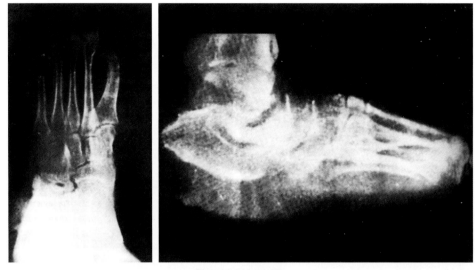

Figs 16.14A and B

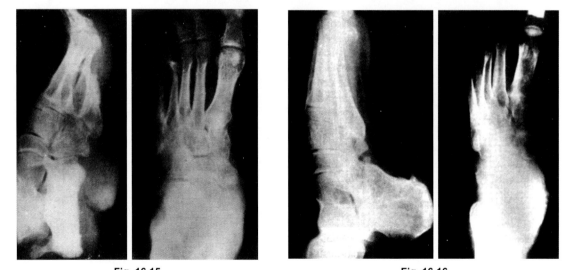

Fig. 16.15   Fig. 16.16

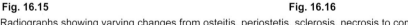
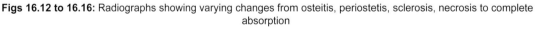

Figs 16.12 to 16.16: Radiographs showing varying changes from osteitis, periostetis, sclerosis, necrosis to complete absorption

b. *Leprous osteitis:* It manifests as an enlarged nutrient foramen, pseudocyst formation, and honey-combing in the distal end of proximal bones.

Nonspecific bone changes result from a combination of sensory loss, trauma and infection. They are comprised of osteitis (hazy bone destruction), concentric bone erosion, absorption of phalanges and osteomyelitis. The destructive lesions occasionally, involve the nasal bone and spine of the maxilla.

Osteoporosis results from prolonged disuse, causing an imbalance between bone absorption by osteoclasts and new bone formation by osteoblasts.

Tendon sheath, tendon and ligaments: The tendons, ligaments and tendon sheaths may get infiltrated replaced by granulation tissue and later heal with contracture and scarring.

SECONDARY CHANGES FOLLOWING NERVE PARALYSIS

Anesthetic Deformity

Hands: The patient is liable to burn his hands due to loss of sensations of temperature and pain. Thus, he continues using his hand inadvertently despite deformity and infection. Infection, in particular, leads to osteomyelitis, tenosynovitis and finally loss of the fingers. Further, with absent tactile sense, the insensitive hand tends to hold objects too tightly for fear of letting them slip. Thus, certain parts of the hand are subjected to high pressure for long periods, causing crush injuries and necrosis of superficial and deep tissue (Figs 16.16 to 16.22).

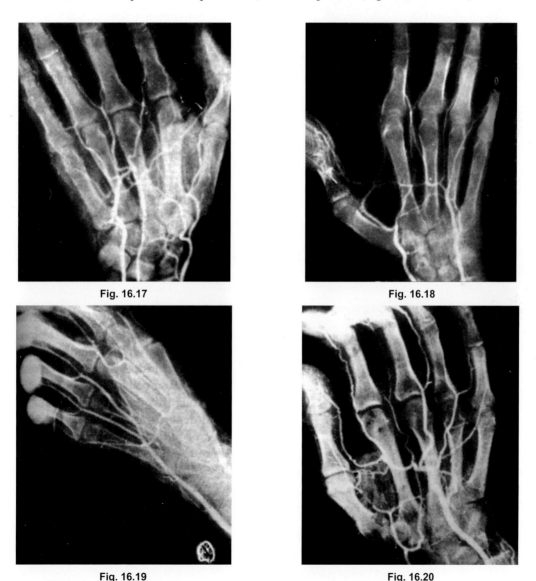

Fig. 16.17   Fig. 16.18

Fig. 16.19   Fig. 16.20

Figs 16.17 to 16.20: Arteriography depicting the status of blood vassals in deformities of the hand

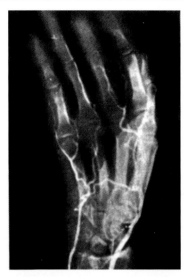

Fig. 16.21: Arteriography changes of narrowing of digital arteries, tortuousity and varying degress of occlusive lesions

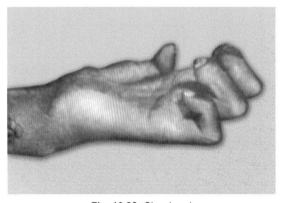

Fig. 16.22: Claw hand

Feet: Leprosy *per se* does not cause trophic ulceration. They develop due to anesthesia of the feet and subsequent recurrent injuries. Similar ulcerations are also seen in peripheral nerve injury, neurosyphilis, diabetic neuropathy and spina bifida. Neglected and unnoticed minor injuries such as cuts, pricks, burns act as portals of entry to microbes, and lead to suppuration and ulceration. A continuous and unrelieved weight-bearing due to constant standing may also be primarily responsible for their development, a process akin to the pathogenesis of bed sores. Walking and not mere standing may be responsible for the pattern of distribution of these ulcers on in the sole. Intrinsic muscles paralysis has

also been incriminated. It has been suggested that interaction of various factors may lead to ulceration of the foot, namely, analgesis, paralysia of intrinsic muscles, stress and strain caused by walking. Also, the replacement of the fibrofatty pad of the foot with scar tissue leads to loss of springing action.

Motor Paralysis and Misuse of Function

Deformity may be caused by motor paralysis distorting the normal position of the hands. This leads to maldistribution of the weight of an object held in the paralytic band. The weight is primarily concentrated on the tips of the fingers of claw hand, instead of getting equally distributed on the palm. There are resultant patches of necrosis and hemorrhages in skin and the bone, which is subsequently replaced by fibrosis, scarring and absorption of the bone culminating ultimately in progressive shortening of the fingers.

Pathogenesis of Larynx Involvement

In lepromatous leprosy, the whole of the upper respiratory tract, from the nose to the bifurcation of the trachea, can be affected. Leprosy of the larynx usually starts in the free margins of the epiglottis as nodular infiltration causing its gradual enlargement. This mass impinges on the airway and obstructs the vocal cords. Grossly, the affected areas have dull-gray nodules. Later, these nodules ulcerate and get covered with exudates. There is a tendency toward healing, scarring and formation of contractures. The vocal cords are usually not involved, until later in the disease.

Pathogenesis of Gynecomastia

The disturbance of liver function, a usual feature in severe lepromatous leprosy, could well be one of the factors in the pathogenesis of gynecomastia. A relative imbalance between the estrogens and androgens, in which estrogen predominates, is also implicated.

Pathogenesis of Blindness in Leprosy

The chronic iridocyclitis from the blood-borne Hansen bacillus gradually leads to the destruction of the ciliary body, and gradual failure of the ocular physiology, which is the most common cause of blindness in leprosy. In a minority, however, the blindness is due to chronic plastic iridocyclitis. Leprous keratitis may also cause some interference with the vision, but this is not serious unless the corneal deposits are very substantial. Other causes of blindness include the neglected cases of lagophthalmos due to involvement of the 7th cranial nerve with or without associated corneal anesthesia, secondary to involvement of the ophthalmic division of the 5th cranial nerve. Both lead to exposure keratitis and corneal ulceration due to trauma and superadded infection, followed by perforation, staphyloma, phthisis bulbi, panophthalmitis and ultimately complete destruction of all structures of the eye.

Prevention and Correction

The deformities and disabilities in leprosy warrant its control, at every level of preventive medicine, as well as its correction, wherever possible, through surgical procedures.

First degree prevention: This essentially should involve the promotion of socioeconomic, health and literacy standard of people throughout the country in general, and in endemic areas in particular. This should also envisage in itself preventing exposure of vulnerable age groups like children, to open cases of leprosy and also BCG vaccination of all family members.

Second degree prevention: It is well known that deformities/disabilities usually develop late in the course of untreated leprosy. Thus, it is implicit that early diagnosis as well as prompt and adequate specific treatment is imperative. Surgical intervention may also be done prevent the deformity. However, if residual anesthesia persists, all patients should be adequately informed to continue to take precautions about the imperceptible thermal or mechanical trauma.

Third degree prevention: Once the patient has developed an irreversible deformity, all efforts should be directed to prevent the conversion of this into a handicap. Hence, the importance of physiotherapist, occupational therapist and also

training of the disabled is in self care. Further, provision of technical aid, educational and enlightening of the public in order to improve community and family attitude toward the disabled and provision of suitable jobs for them is also essential.

▮ DEFORMITY CORRECTIVE MEASURES

Physiotherapy

Different strengthening exercises should be given to improve muscles power and tone. Proper footwear has to be devised and individualized, to prevent trauma to the anesthetic foot. Microcellular rubber footwear effectively serves the purpose. Wax bath, hydrotherapy and massage should also be given with the objective to improve blood circulation. Passive stretching exercises improve and maintain joint mobility further, exercises can be instituted which will increase the range of movements. Assistance in correction of deformities can additionally be achieved by application of plaster of paris (POP) splints. The various splints used are circular, thumb-web, gutter, functional dynamic and walking plaster splints.

Reconstructive surgery for hands: Claw-hand can be corrected by providing a new muscle attachment to the affected fingers. This can be achieved through any of the many muscle transfer operations used in the past. Flexor digitorum superficialis (Bunnell's operation), extensor carpi radialis (Brands' operation), extensor indices and digit minimi (Fowlers' operation), palmaris longus and flexor carpi radialis all can be utilized for the purpose, thus restoring the function of the lumbricals. Flexor digitorum sublimes of the ring finger can be utilized in cases of thumb paralysis. If the finger(s) are too stiff to be mobilized by tendon transfer, arthrodesis in the functional position can be done.

Reconstructive surgery of the foot: For the correction of foot-drop, the unaffected muscles at the back of the leg can be utilized for transfer operations. Of them, tibialis posterior tendon is usually used. In cases where this cannot be done, footwear with toe-raising spring/straps must be provided for the patient. Mild cases of claw toes should be corrected by closed tenotomy and plastic casts. In advanced cases, interphalangeal arthrodesis in functional position is indicated. The management of trophic ulcers includes complete bed rest, antibiotic administration, eusol dressing and walking plaster cast. However, if these measures fail or if the ulcer is too big, skin grafting after debridement may be required.

Reconstructive surgery of the face: Lagophthalmos can be surgically corrected through tarsorrhaphy or temporalis muscles transfer. Nose bridge depression can be corrected by simple bone or cartilage graft, postnasal epithelial inlay or by tube pedicle rhinoplasty.

Reconstructive surgery of gynecomastia: Cosmetic correction of the embarrassing gynecomastia can be done using Webster's operation.

▌RECOMMENDED READING

1. Anonymous. WHO, Disability prevention and rehabilition. Technical Report Series No. 668, 1981.
2. Brand PW. Treatment of leprosy II. The role of surgery. *N Engl J Med*. 1956;254:64-67.
3. Enna CD. The deformities of leprosy. In: Surgical rehabilittion in leprosy. McDowell F, Enna CD Eds, Williams nd wilkins, Battimore, 1974.
4. Sehgal VN, Sharma PK. Pattern of deformities/disabilities in urban leprosy. *Indian J Lepr*. 1985;57:183-192.
5. Sehgal VN, Srivastava G, HD deformities and disabilities: current status. Part 1. *The Star*. 1988;47:10-13.
6. Sehgal VN, Srivastava G, HD Deformities and disabilities: current status. *The Star*. 1988;47:8-11, 16.
7. Smith WC, Parkhe SM. Disability assessment as a measure of progress in leprosy control. *Lepr Rev*. 1986;57:251-259.

Therapy of Leprosy

Since the introduction of dapsone three decades ago for the treatment of leprosy, several of its derivatives, namely, glucosulfone sodium (Promine), sulfoxone sodium (Diasone sodium), sulphetrone sodium (Solapsone), thiazole sulfone (Primizole) were used. But due to inconvenient administration and side-effects, their use has largely been relegated in favor of dapsone—the parent compound.

DAPSONE

Dapsone-4: 4' diaminodiphenylsulfone (DDS). It has remained the drug of choice for its treatment. It has stood the test of time, and possesses certain advantages. It is primarily administered orally and is inexpensive, having low risk of toxicity, and possesses high degree of clinical effectiveness with infrequent relapse. Following is its structure.

It is effective against *Mycobacterium leprae*. Its effective estimated sensitivity is 0.02 μg/ml in micro-organisms recovered from untreated patients. It is bacteriostatic. The organisms may become resistant to the drug during therapy.

Its probable mode of action consists of preventing the utilization of para-aminobenzoic acid (PABA), which is essential for the growth of certain organisms including *mycobacterium leprae*—an action similar to that of sulfonamides.

Dapsone is slowly and almost completely absorbed from the body fluid, and is present in all tissues. It gets accumulated in the skin, muscles, liver and kidneys and also in the circulation for a long time because of intestinal re-absorption from the bile. It is acetylated in the liver and the degree of acetylation is genetically determined. The minimal effective level of dapsone in the blood is 0.15 mg per 100 ml. The drug is largely excreted through the kidneys in the urine.

Dapsone (dapson, cryosulfone, novosulfone, siosulfone) is available as tablets containing 100 mg. It is given by the oral route. The dose is calculated as 6–10 mg/kg body weight per week in daily divided doses. It is effective against all types of leprosy and clinical improvement is seen practically in every case. Younger the patient and earlier the treatment is started, betters the therapeutic response. The mucosal lesions, namely, oral, nasal, pharyngeal and laryngeal nodules, infiltration and ulcerations regress faster (6 months to 1 year), while skin manifestations require longer period (1 to 3 years). Generally, there is a rapid clinical than bacteriological improvement.

Untoward effects: Anorexia, nausea and vomiting may be observed. Instances of headache, nervousness, insomnia, blurred vision, paraesthesia, hamaturia may be recorded. Pruritus and drug fever may appear. Psychosis may rarely be seen, especially with high dosage. Skin rashes of various types including erythema multiforme, Stevens'-Johnson syndrome, fixed drug eruption may also be encountered. Hepatitis with attending symptoms may infrequently be seen.

Dapsone may be responsible for precipitating or triggering the reactions in leprosy—erythema nodosum leprosum—in lepromatous and borderline leprosy and the reaction in other types. These reactions are probably an evidence of activity of the drug. Sulfone syndrome, characterized by fever, malaise, exfoliative dermatitis, jaundice, hepatic necrosis, lymphadenopathy, methemoglobinemia, anemia may envisage the immediate withdrawal of the drug.

Varying degree of hemolysis is a common associated feature of dapsone therapy, but development of hemolytic anemia is usual. It may develop either because of deficiency of glucose-6-phosphate dehydrogenase, disorder of bone marrow and/or because of high dosage, methemoglobinemia with Heinz bodies formation may occur.

Acedapsone

It is diacetyldiaminodiphenyl sulfone (DADDS)—a diacetyl derivative of dapsone. It is administered parentrally as a repository preparation. Its therapeutic properties are similar to those of dapsone. It is being used only as a drug under trial, for it is not freely available. It is used mainly for domiciliary line of treatment. Continuous effective levels of dapsone are maintained in the blood for a period of 75 days. In view of the fact that its blood level is not adequate and effective, emergence of dapsone resistant strains of *Mycobacterium leprae* is being feared.

Amithiozone

It is derivative of thiosemicarbazone-4 acetyl-aminoaldehyde thiosemicarbazone with the following structure.

$$CH_3-\underset{\underset{O}{\|}}{C}-NH-\langle\!\bigcirc\!\rangle-CH=N-NH-\underset{\underset{S}{\|}}{C}-NH_2$$

It is effective against *Mycobacterium leprae*. It is bacteriostatic. It appears to exert a greater effect in tuberculoid than on lepromatous and borderline leprosy. *Mycobacterium leprae* develops resistance to these agents in the early stage.

It is well absorbed from the gastrointestinal tract, and a large amount is excreted through the urine. It is metabolized rapidly. Its exact mode of action is not known, however, it is likely that, metabolites of these compounds may possess antibacterial activity.

Amithiozone (Thiacetazone): It is available in 25 mg, 50 mg and 150 mg tablets for oral use. The initial dose is 50 mg per day, for one to two weeks, after which the daily quantity is gradually increased to a maximum of 200 mg. The efficacy of the drug increases when it is given in a single dose. Its effect is marked only in first year followed by a slower rate of improvement in the second year and the occurrence of relapse in the third year. The drug can be used effectively only for one to two years. Hence, it is a poor substitute for dapsone; even then, it is being used as a substitute for dapsone in developing countries because of its low cost.

■ CLOFAZIMINE

It is 3-(p-chloro-anilino-)-10–(p-chlorophenyl) 2, 10-dihydro-3-(Isopropyl amino)-phenazine.

It exerts a bacteriostatic and mildly bactericidal effect on *M. leprae*. Clofazimine also possesses anti-inflammatory, immunomodulatory and steroid sparing properties. It combines with DNA to inhibit its template function. It also inhibits the migration and proliferation of white blood corpuscles *in vitro* and *in vivo*. It is absorbed rather slowly. The unchanged active substance reaches a peak plasma concentration 8 to 12 hours after a single oral dose. Administration of the drug with food increases its bioavailability. The half life for the elimination of unchanged clofazimine from the plasma in healthy subjects is 8–11 days, following both single and repeated doses. Consequently, steady-state plasma concentrations are not attained until after 30–40 days. Clofazimine is strongly lipophilic and accumulates in the fatty tissues and in the macrophages of the reticuloendothelial system. Patients who undergo long-term treatment with clofazimine accumulate it in the subcutaneous fat, in the mesenteric lymphnodes, in the bile and gallbladder, in the adrenals, spleen, small intestine, liver muscles, bones and skin but never in the brain. Clofazimine is excreted mainly in the feces.

Clofazimine is employed in combination with dapsone and rifampicin for the treatment of multibacillary leprosy (BT, BB, BL, LL) and is administered as 300 mg supervised dose every month and 50 mg daily self-administered. It is also used in the management of type I (reversal) and type II (ENL) reactions where it may be administered in a dose of 200–300 mg daily. It should be taken at meal times or together with milk. It is contraindicated in those hypersensitive to clofazimine. Leprosy patients suffering from abdominal pain and diarrhea, as well as those with liver or kidney damage should, if possible, be not treated with clofazimine. If the gastrointestinal symptoms develop during the treatment, the dosage should be rduced or interval between the dosage prolonged. In the event of persistent diarrhea or vomiting, the patient should be hospitalized. Clofazimine should be used with caution during the first trimester of pregnancy. It crosses the placental barrier and causes temporary discoloration of new born infants. The active substance also passes into the breast milk. Reddish to dark brown discoloration of hair, conjunctiva, cornea and lacrimal fluid as well as of the sweat, sputum, urine and feces may occur. The discoloration is reversible, though it may take some months after the cessation of the treatment. Dryness of the skin, ichthyosis, pruritus, photosensitivity, acne form eruptions, nonspecific rashes, nausea, vomiting, abdominal pain, diarrhea, anorexia, loss of weight and eosinophilic enteropathy are its other side effects.

RIFAMPICIN

This is a semi synthetic derivative of rifamycin-B, isolated from *Streptomyces mediteranei*. It is the most potent bactericidal antileprosy drug. A single dose of 600 mg kills 99.9 per cent of the lepra bacilli within a few days, and thus speedily renders a patient of multibacillary leprosy noninfectious. Rifampicin acts by inhibiting DNA-depends RNA polymerase, thus suppressing bacterial ribonucleic acid synthesis. Their minimum inhibitory concentration is 0.3 µg/ml.

It is absorbed in its entirety from the gastrointestinal tract, and attains a peak plasma concentration 2–3 hours after ingestion on an empty stomach. It has plasma half life of 2–3 hours. Rifampicin passes in therapeutically active concentration in body fluids and tissues. The bulk of it is excreted in the bile and only a small proportion in the urine.

It is used in the treatment of pauci-and multibacillary leprosy as a part component of multidrug therapy (MDT). It is administered in the supervised monthly dosage of 600 mg for six months in cases of paucibacillary leprosy (I,TT) and for at least 2 years or till smear, negativity is achieved in multibacillary leprosy (BT, BB, BL, LL). Persons weighing less than 35 kg should be administered 450 mg of rifampicin in leprosy is attributed to its being potent bactericidal, related to the very long generation time of lepra bacilli. Thus once monthly single rifampicin dose represents a substantial cost reduction in the treatment of leprosy and ensures administration of the drug under supervision. However, it may predispose to bacterial resistance and 'persisters' which are responsible for treatment failure and relapse, respectively. Thus, to overcome this, the American regimen recommends daily administration of the drug. It is available as 150 mg and 300 mg capsules.

Rifampicin is contraindicated in those hypersensitive to refamycins. The adverse effects of rifampicin occur in less than 5 percent of the patients. It is a bright reddish-brown colored substance and cause reddish discoloration of the urine, sputum and lacrimal fluids. It causes gastrointestinal disturbances like disorder of hepatic functions with mild transient elevation of transaminases, jaundice and hepatitis. However, mild gastrointestinal side effects do not necessitate discontinuation of the therapy. It may cause leukopenia, thrombocytopenia, osteomalacia, psychosis, weakness, ataxia and dizziness. It may also cause pemphigus vulgaris and Stevens-Johnson syndrome and precipitate porphyria cutanea tarda. The intermittent therapy may be associated with the flu-like syndrome. However, it is rare in leprosy patients. Rifampicin stimulates hepatic microsomal enzymes which increase the metabolic degradation of steroids. Thus, daily administration of rifampicin may reduce the effectiveness of the steroids.

ETHIONAMIDE

It is a drug with a chemical structure closely related to that of isoniazid. It has a potent bactericidal action against *M. leprae*. This action is faster than the full dosage of dapsone but slower than rifampicin.

It is believed to act by inhibiting the protein synthesis in the cell. Resistance may develop both *in vivo* and *in vitro*. Such organisms show cross resistance to thiosemicarbazone.

It is absorbed fairly rapidly from the gastrointestinal tract (GIT). It is widely and rapidly distributed in the body tissues. The metabolic fate of the drug is not known. Less than 1 percent of the drug is excreted in the active form in urine.

Ethionamide is available as 125 mg and 250 mg tablets. It is usually administered in the dosage of 5 mg/kg/day. An average sized adults requires 375 mg of ethionamide every day.

Gastrointestinal disturbance occurs in a majority of patients and include metallic taste in the mouth,

ptyalism, nausea, vomiting, anorexia and diarrhea. To minimize the GIT irritation, the drug may be given as a single dose after the meals at bedtime. Hepatitis is observed in 5 percent of the cases. Allergic manifestation include skin rashes and alopecia. Occasionally serious manifestations like postural hypotension and anaphylactic shock may result. It may also cause impotence, menorrhagia, hypothyroidism, gynaecomastia and psychosis. The control of diabetes mellitus is made difficult as it may precipitate hypoglycemia.

CHEMOTHERAPY OF LEPROSY

Earlier, treatment of leprosy was restricted to dapsone monotherapy. It predisposed to the emergence of secondary and subsequent primary dapsone resistant bacilli. In order to check the spread of drug resistant mutants, WHO recommended the multidrug therapy with the objective of (1) to cure the patient (2) to interrupt the transmission of the infection in the community (3) to stall the emergence of drug resistant mutants (4) to prevent the deformities. WHO favoured classification of the patient into pauci- and multibacillary based on the bacterial index (BI) recorded by the slit-skin smear examination. They were considered paucibacillary (PB) if BI was less than 2 and multibacillary (MB) when BI was 2 or more. PB included indeterminate (I), tuberculoid (TT) and borderline tuberculoid (BT); wile MB included borderline-borderline (BB), borderline lepromatous (BL) and lepromatous leprosy (LL). However, recently WHO has modified its criteria for treatment. All smear positive patients are considered multibacillary (BT, BB, BL and LL), whereas smear negative patients are paucibacillary indeterminate (I), tubeculoid (TT).

A short course chemotherapy for 6 months is recommended for paucibacillary patients and it is administered to:

1. All freshly diagnosed cases of paucibacillary leprosy.
2. All dapsone treated paucibacillary patients who have relapsed.
3. Paucibacillary patients who are currently on treatment with dapsone, but have not yet completed 2 years (Table 17.1).

Table 17.1: Chemotherapy for paucibacillary (PB) leprosy

Clinical Group	Drugs	Dosage and Mode of administration	Duration
1*, TT	Rifampicin	600 mg once monthly supervised	6 doses of rifampicin to be administered in maximum of nine months
	Dapsone	100 mg daily self-administered	

*An endeavor should be made to diagnose cases of indeterminate leprosy (I) beyond doubt. For this clinical, bacteriological, histopathological and immunological parameters are taken into account. An attempt is made to demonstrate AFB on hematoxylin-eosin stained serial sections. If possible, lepromin and FLA-ABS should be done. The result is interpreted as:
1. Diagnosis is in doubt—prudent to keep patient under observation
2. Lepromin +ve, FLA=Abs +ve, should be treated as PB.
3. Lepromin –ve, FLA-Abs +ve, should be treated as MB.

Table 17.2: Chemotherapy for multibacillary (MB) leprosy

Clinical Group	Drugs	Dosage and Mode of administration	Duration
BT, BB, BL, LL	Rifampicin	600 mg once monthly supervised	2 Years or preferably till smear negativity
	Dapsone	100 mg daily self-administered	
	Clofazimine	300 mg supervised every month and 50 mg daily self-administered	

The treatment is stopped after 6 months. As the bacterial load is low (10^6), it is perceived that the adequate CMI will help in the spontaneous resolution of the granuloma and also contain the persisters.

The proposed chemotherapeutic regimen for multibacillary (MB) leprosy is recommended for (Table 17.2):
1. Freshly diagnosed MB cases.
2. Patients who have responded satisfactorily to previous dapsone monotherapy.
3. Patients who have not responded satisfactorily to previous dapsone monotherapy.
4. Patients who have relapsed after cessation of dapsone monotherapy.

The exact time required to achieve the cure is not known. However, the treatment is recommended for a minimum of 2 years, and if possible till smear negativity.

Although the above regimen is cheap, ensures better patients' compliance, and pulses ensure the drug, yet it may predispose to:
- Drug resistant leprosy
- Persisters
- Relapse.

RECOMMENDED READING

1. Anonymous. Adverse reactions to dapsone. *Lancet*. 1981;2:184-185.
2. Anonymous. Expert committee on leprosy. Sixth Technical Report Series No. 768, WHO, Geneva 14, 1988.
3. Anonymous. WHO study group. Chemotherapy of leprosy for control programmes, Geneva; WHO Technical Report Series NO. 675. 1982.
4. Jopling WH. Side effects of antileprosy drugs in common use. *Lepr Rev*. 1983;54:261-270.
5. Yawalkar SJ, Vischer WA. Lamprene in leprosy: basic information, 2nd edn, Pharma Division, Ciba-Geigy LTD, Basic, Switzerland, 1984.

18

Newer Antileprosy Drugs

Ideally a new antileprosy drug should possess (1) strong bacterial action against *M. leprae* without antagonism to available drugs (2) safe and well tolerated by the patient (3) easy to administer orally in a single daily dose.

FLUOROQUINOLONES

The fluoroquinolones inhibit bacterial DNA gyrase, a target which has not yet been exploited in leprosy. Pefloxacin and ofloxacin display potent bactericidal activity against *M. leprae*. Both the drugs have demonstrated rapid bactericidal activity by serial mouse foot pad inoculation. The rifampicin resistant mutants are killed by fluoroquinolones by 22 doses of either ofloxacin or pefloxacin. Thus the combination of ofloxacin (400 mg daily/pefloxacin (800 mg daily) and rifampicin may considerably shorten the duration of multidrug therapy.

Recently, seven new fluoroquinolones, AT-4140, OPC-17100, OPC=17066, PD-117596, PD-124816, PD-127391 and WIN-57273 have been demonstrated to be more active against *M. leprae in vitro*.

MINOCYCLINE

Among the tetracyclines, minocycline is unique, and is active against *M. leprae*. Its lipophilic property allows it to penetrate the cell wall of *M. leprae*. Minocycline is a safe drug and clinical trials are being conducted to evaluate the bactericidal activity of 100 mg of minocycline daily in previously untreated lepromatous patients.

MACROLIDES

Several semi-synthetic macrolides including azithromycin, clarithromycin, roxithromycin, M-119-31 and M-119-49 have been evaluated for bactericidal activity against *M. leprae*. Roxithromycin was unable to inhibit multiplication of *M. leprae* in mouse foot pad, whereas clarithromycin demonstrated strong bactericidal activity *M. leprae*. Clarithromycin is well tolerated and clinical trials are being undertaken with different doses of clarithromycin among previously untreated lepromatous patients.

PHENAZINE

Clofazimine, a phenazine derivative is one of the components of MDT for multibacillary patients. It has bactericidal activity against *M. leprae*. Also it has anti-inflammatory, immunomodulatory and steroid-sparing action. Coloration of the skin is the major limitation. Recently a series of phenazine derivatives have been synthesized without the preceding effect. Though most of the derivatives are active *in vitro* against *M. leprae*, however, the results *in vitro* are not encouraging. It may be attributed to low lipophilicity of such compounds.

Drugs related to existing MDT with antimycobacterial properties

1. Rifamycin: Rifampicin; Rifabutin; Rifapentine; T9; and KRM-1648.
2. Phenazine: Clofazimine (B-663); B-4071; B-4087; B-746; and B-4100.
3. Dihydrofolate reductase inhibitor: Dapsonε²; Brodimoprim; Epiroprim; and K-130.

Newer classes of antileprosy drugs

1. Fluoroquinolone: Ofloxacin; Pefloxacin; Sparfloxacin; Levofloxacin; Temofloxacin; Clinafloxacin; and Moxifloxacin.
2. Tetracycline: Minocycline.
3. Macrolide: Clarithromycin; and Telithromycin (ketolide).

RIFAMYCIN DERIVATIVES

In the footpad of mine, strong bactericidal activities have been demonstrated by several rifamycin derivatives including rifabutin (LM-427), rifapentine (DL-473) and R-76-1. All these derivatives are more effective on a weight for weight basis than rifampicin. However, their activity against rifampicin resistant strain of *M. leprae* has not yet been confirmed.

Some newer antileprosy drugs which are being worked up for use are being tabulated.

RECOMMENDED READING

1. Bhattacharya SN, Sehgal VN. Reappraisal of drifting scenario of Leprosy multidrug therapy: new approach proposed for the the new millennium. *Int J Dermatol*. 2002;41:321-326.
2. Dhople AM. Search for newer leprosy drugs. *Indian J Lepr*. 2000;72:5-20.
3. Ji B, Grosset JH. Recent advances in the chemotherapy of leprosy. *Lepr Rev*. 1990;61:313-329.
4. Wayne LG, Sramek HA. Metronidazole is bactericidal to dormant cells of *Mycobacterium tuberculosis*. *Antimicrob Agents Chemother*. 1994; 38:2054-2058.

Basic Requirements for Implementation of Multidrug Therapy

In 1982, the World Health Organization (WHO), officially recommended that leprosy should be treated with multidrug therapy (MDT). Experience in using the WHO recommended MDT regimens have shown that they are effective, safe and acceptable to patients and field staff.

However, only 39.5 percent of the 4.3 million leprosy patients registered for chemotherapy at the end of 1988 were on MDT, while a cumulative number of one million patients had completed treatment with MDT. Apparently, far too many leprosy patients do not have access to the benefits of MDT. To a great extent, this regrettable situation can be attributed to the fact that in many countries the health services cannot fulfill the complex and demanding requirements for the introduction of MDT which were identified some eight years ago.

A working group of the ILEP Medical Commissions' Leprosy Expert Discipline, in which program managers from various-parts of the world participated, met in Brussels in September 1989 in order to review these requirements and to formulate recommendations which are appropriate to the real field situation in many leprosy endemic countries. The recommendations were endorsed by the Medical Commission in December 1989 and were slightly adapted after the interface Meeting of the ILE member associations and the Medical Commissions in June 1990. They represent the consensus of the members of the working group and the Medical Commission.

These recommendation concern basic rather than optimal requirements, which are intended especially for those program which otherwise could not implement MDT.

The following are the suggested recommendations.

INTRODUCTION

The current strategy for leprosy control is early diagnosis and the provision of effective chemotherapy in order to cure the patient, to interrupt transmission and to prevent leprosy related disabilities.

At present, regular and complete course with multidrug therapy (MDT) of all known leprosy cases and early diagnosed new cases is the best available effective approach to achieve leprosy control and its use must be the top priority for leprosy control program. Using this approach will decrease the need for social, psychological and economic rehabilitation of the leprosy patient.

Until now on the global scale the coverage of MDT has been too slow. There has been hesitation to use MDT especially because the requirements proposed for its introduction were too demanding for the health services in many leprosy-endemic countries. In order to assist ILEP members to quickly expand the coverage of MDT, in their own projects as well as those of national and local governments, the basis rather that the optimal requirements which should be met, before MDT is implemented, have been identified as follows.

THE MDT REGIMEN

- MDT should be given to all patients in need of chemotherapy.
- In principle, there is no longer a place for dapsone monotherapy. Where dapsone mono-therapy is used, every effort must be made to transfer the patients to MDT.
- The WHO recommended MDT regimens for multibacillary (MB) and paucibacillary (PB) leprosy. They are recommended for routine field conditions. Experience has shown that they are effective, safe and operationally feasible. They are acceptable to patients and field staff.

This does not imply that where some countries have already introduced other multidrug regimens which have proven to be equally effective and safe, that these are to be changed.

2.4 Experience with the WHO MDT regimens has shown that 24 monthly doses in 36 months for MB patients and 6 monthly doses in 9 months for PB patients, is adequate, thus continuation of treatment beyond these periods is not necessary in the vast majority of the cases.

The available evidence indicates that the risk of relapse after MDT is low. Moreover, as it is always possible to adequately retreat relapsed cases, the possibility of relapse after treatment should be accepted.

- The principle of monthly supervised intake of drugs should be adhered to and, ideally, supervision should be done at the peripheral health service and by a health worker. However, if a health worker is unavailable, a village leader, teacher, family member could be given this responsibility.

In particular, cases such as migrant workers, inaccessible roads due to the rainy season, the patient could be entrusted with more than one month's supply of blister calendar packs is indicated.

- The following are reasons for stopping MDT:
- Severe liver disease,
- Severe toxic/allergic side-effects to the drugs.

In leprosy patients, suffering from tuberculosis, the treatment for these diseases should be given simultaneously.

THE BASIC REQUIREMENT WHICH MUST BE MET BEFORE IMPLEMENTING MDT

Multidrug therapy (MDT) can be introduced into and successfully implemented in all existing health infrastructures in leprosy-endemic countries, if the following basic requirements are fulfilled:

Political and Professional Commitment

In principle, commitment at all administrative levels is essential to expand the coverage of MDT.

In practice, the commitment of one or two key professional individuals in the health service to introduce MDT at a local level is the basic requirement.

A Plan of Action

This can be a simple statement of objectives, main activities with targets and timetable, a statement of finances needed and information on who is responsible for the allocation of resources.

Operational Guidelines

This can be a single document which includes information on:
- Job descriptions,
- Supervisory schedules,
- Criteria for the diagnosis and classification of patients,
- Criteria for the selection of patients for MDT, this includes criteria for screening old patients currently on register,
- Treatment regimens,
- Management of patients during treatment including periodicity of examination, absentee tracing, prevention of disability and management of complications (including referral procedure),
- Procedure at release from treatment,
- Recording and reporting of patients data.

Competent Staff

Staff responsible for leprosy control should be able to diagnose leprosy, treat patients and give health education on regularity of drug intake and disability preventing to patients. Their training should be task-oriented according to appropriate job descriptions.

Well trained paramedical workers can diagnose leprosy, give treatment with MDT and give adequate health education. As treatment has a fixed duration the paramedical worker can release patients from treatment. Thus, it is not absolutely necessary for every patient to be seen by a doctor.

At the regional/provincial and/or district levels, staff with adequate knowledge and skills in the field of management of leprosy control should be available for supervision, training and referral.

Availability of Drugs

There must be an adequate logistical system to guarantee a secure and uninterrupted drug supply.

Collection of Basic Data

The following is the minimum data required:
- Number of patients registered for chemotherapy (MB/PB).
- Number of patients registered for MDT (MB/PB).
- Proportion of patients who have successfully completed MDT within the required time period (MB/PB).
- Although the availability of the following data is not a prerequisite for the introduction of MDT, collection of this information is recommended in order to monitor the effectiveness of case finding, and disability prevention activities.
- Proportion of cases with diabilities (grade 2) among newly detected.
- Proportion of patients who developed new disabilities among those on register MDT.

Case Detection Activities

With the introduction of good quality service, voluntary self-reporting should be the basis of conducting cases. Active case finding can be limited to the examination of the patients' contacts.

This can also be a useful occasion also to improve the motivation of the patient through fostering the support of the family.

Diagnosis

The vast majority of leprosy patients who report voluntarily to the health services can be diagnosed by using clinical skills only.

With the application of well-defined criteria, a number of programs, base the classification into MB and PB leprosy on clinical findings alone. (To help field programs, the ILEP Medical Commission intends to convene a working group to define the most appropriate criteria for this purpose).

If there is doubt about the classification of leprosy, the MDT regimen as applicable for MB leprosy should be given.

Laboratory Services

Skin smear examination is necessary in the diagnosis of early lepromatous cases and is useful in monitoring the classification which was made on clinical grounds. Therefore, it is recommended that reliable skin smear services should be established.

In practice, however, skin smear services in most programs are not reliable. As already discussed (*vide supra*), almost all patients can be diagnosed using clinical skills only. The availability of skin-smear services is thus not an absolute pre-requisite for starting MDT.

Care Activities

Early diagnosis and adequate treatment with MDT are the most important means of preventing disabilities.

Whilst the early detection of neuritis and the treatment of reactions are extremely important, the lack of this service should not be a barrier to the introduction of MDT.

The main responsibility for the prevention of new increasing disabilities should be given to the patient.

Health education in self care practices should be given to those patients at risk of developing disabilities.

Though the early detection of neuritis and the treatment of reactions are extremely important, the provision of this care is not an absolute requirement to the introduction of MDT. However, it is strongly recommended that these services should be established as soon as possible.

Surveillance after MDT Treatment

It is recommended that passive surveillance only is carried out. Each patient should be aware at the time of release from treatment of the need to contact the health services if problems are experienced.

Rehabilitation Services

The availability of rehabilitation services although important and desirable is not a prerequisite for introducing MDT. However, if rehabilitation services exist for the physically or socially handicapped, every effort should be made to make these services available for leprosy patients as well.

THE FRAMEWORK FOR IMPLEMENTATION OF MDT

ILEP members should aim at the implementation of MDT through the General Health Services (Based on the primary health care approach). This would give a wider and more comprehensive coverage and provide greater continuity of service. Where this is not yet possible, vertical services may still be appropriate but consideration should be given to combining the leprosy service with other vertical health programs as a transition towards full integration. Within the integrated program a specialized component should be available at the more central levels for supervision, training and referral. ILEP members' can play a crucial role in expanding the coverage of MDT.

RECOMMENDED READING

1. Anonymous. Basic requirement for implementation of multidrug therapy—ILEP Medical Bulletin. *Lepr Rev.* 1990;61:386-390.

20

Drug-resistance, Persisters and Relapse

Drug-resistance in *Mycobacterium leprae* is a crucial topic to which pointed attention has been focused recently. Before the advent of multidrug therapy (MDT), it was a frequent occurrence because of conventional monotherapy with diaminodiphenyl sulfone (DDS). Reports of resistance to other drugs as well, namely, rifampicin and clofazimine are now available. It may pose a potential threat to the effective control of the disease in years to come, because dissemination of the disease to other healthy individuals may be difficult to arrest with currently available drugs. Hence, it is essential to recognize the situation before it emerges as a threatening problem.

Drug-resistance may be either secondary or primary. Secondary drug-resistance in *M. Leprae* is usually induced by drugs, whereas no such exposure to drugs may be present in primary drug-resistance. Slit-skin smear examination and study of the morphology of the organisms may be vital to identify such cases. Clinical criteria may be important instruments for early diagnosis and treatment of drug-resistant leprosy.

1. The initial classification of the disease into multibacillary and paucibacillary should be clearly defined on the basis of slit-skin smear examination. Multibacillary cases (BT, BB, BL, and LL) are more prone to develop drug-resistance as compared with paucibacillary cases (I, TT).

2. It is important to maintain a record of the administration of antileprosy drugs in detail regarding monotherapy with diaminodiphenyl sulphone, its dosage as well as the regularity of treatment. The same holds true for rifampicin and clofazimine. Furthermore, the duration of treatment is also important.

3. Following the administration of antileprosy drugs for a period ranging from 6–12 months, a perceptible amelioration in the clinical symptoms and signs is recorded, after which the improvement is stalled or deterioration sets in. It may be possible to document this, based on erythema or edema or both, of the macule/plaque, thickening or tenderness or both of the nerves supplying the plaques and ultimate demonstration of *M. leprae* through Zeihl-Neelsen stained slit-skin smears.

4. Slit-skin smear examination is a vital factor in finalizing the diagnosis of drug-resistant leprosy. This is achieved by detailed study of the morphological features of the lepra bacilli. Resistant *M. leprae* shows solid uniform staining, the sides of the bacilli are parallel with rounded ends, and its length is five times its width. Morphological index (MI) will be more than what it was earlier. MI determination is an important laboratory procedure and it should be carefully undertaken. It is determined by counting the number of both regularly and irregularly stained bacilli in the slit-skin

smear. Only bacilli showing uniform staining throughout their length should be considered regularly stained. The count should preferably be of 100 or more organisms in field, picked at random. MI is calculated as the number of regularly stained bacilli per hundred of the organisms examined, e.g.

Number of bacilli counted = 100
Number of regularly stained = 10 bacilli
Morphological index = 10 percent

5. Should the facilities for inoculation of the bacteria in hybrid, thymectomized irradiated or nude mice exist, that may ultimately confirm the diagnosis of drug-resistance.

The prevalent multidrug therapy for pauci–and multibacillary leprosy may, therefore, have implicit limitations as far as dosage, mode of administration, and duration are concerned. The regimen as advocated by the US Public Health

Service, therefore, needs careful consideration for adoption. It has merit, and endeavors to be rational and saves a couple of drugs for managing drug-resistant leprosy. A short resume of it is outlined above (Table 20.1).

In addition to drug-resistant leprosy following drug therapy, 'persisters' and relapse may complicate leprosy control. It is, therefore, imperative to comprehend these terms. The persisters are viable, fully drug-susceptible forms of *Mycobacterium leprae* which are able to survive for many years in the patient despite the presence of adequate bactericidal concentration of an anti-leprosy drug. They are regarded as physiologically dormant forms favoring certain sites like the peripheral nerves, smooth and striated muscles and viscera. Such viable and fully drug-sensitive strains may be isolated from the patient who has received treatment for 10–12 years with dapsone and for five years with rifampicin. They can survive a period of

Table 20.1: US Public Health Service Regimen			
A. Paucibacillary (PB)			
1. Drugs	DDS + Followed by Rifampin	DDS	
2. Daily dose	100 mg 600 mg	100 mg	
3. Duration	6 months	3 years	5 years
4. Groups	PB (I, TT, BT)	I, TT	BT
B. Multibacillary (MB)			
1. Drugs	DDS + Followed by Rifampin	DDS	
2. Daily dose	100 mg 600 mg	100 mg	
3. Duration	3 years	10 years	Life
4. Groups	MB (BB,BL,LL)	BB	BL, LL
C. Dapsone resistant M. leprae			
1. Drugs	Clofazimine + Followed by Rifampin	Clofazimine	
2. Daily dose	50 mg 600 mg	50 mg	
3. Duration	3 years	Indefinitely	
4. Groups	MB (BB,BL,LL)	MB (BB,BL,LL)	
OR			
1. Drugs	Rifampin + Ethionamide		
2. Daily dose	600 mg + 250 mg		
3. Duration	Indefinitely		
4. Groups	MB (BB,BL,LL)		

over 20 years and are responsible for relapse in a proportion of cases.

Relapse/reactivation is encountered both in multibacillary (MB) and in paucibacillary (PB) patients, who were administered multidrug therapy (MDT) as per the recommendation of the World Health Organization. The relapses are infrequent in paucibacillary leprosy, because of the low bacterial load and the short course of treatment. The patients were followed for regression of clinical and histological signs of the activity of the disease. Regression of clinical signs is important in field work and is indicated by reduction of edema or erythema or both, of the cutaneous lesions and thickening or tenderness or both, of the cutaneous nerves supplying or feeding the lesions. The patient is free of signs and symptoms of the disease for a considerable period of time, after which lesions reappear on a few previously affected areas; the entire area or part of it may be involved. This is enforced by reappearance of thickening or tenderness or both of the previously affected nerves, which had become quiescent following adequate treatment. The reappearance of activity is insidious and may occur long after the stoppage of treatment. Histopathology and lepromin reaction conform to the classification of the previous episode, inferring thereby that during the relapse, the classification does not change. Furthermore, these cases show successful response to only multidrug therapy (MDT).

Relapse in paucibacillary cases may, therefore, be differentiated from that of Type-I (lepra) reaction, the details of which are given in Table 20.3. Furthermore, it is also imperative to appreciate the criteria for differentiating relapse from drug-resistant leprosy (Table 20.2).

Table 20.2: Drug-resistant leprosy and relapse

Drug-Resistant Leprosy	Relapse
1. Secondary or primary drug-resistant *M. leprae*	'Persisters'
2. Initial amelioration followed by subsequent halt/deterioration during MDT	Recurrence after release from MDT surveillance
3. Appearance of new lesions in addition to extension of the existing ones	Reappearance of activity in part or whole of the previous lesion(s)
4. Progressive thickening, tenderness or both, of unaffected nerves	Quiescent nerve(s) again become thickened and tender
5. Increased bacterial index (BI) and declining lepromin reaction	BI and lepromin reactions are uncharged
6. May downgrade from BT→BB→BL→LL	Original classification does not change
7. Bacilli are resistant to one or more antileprosy drugs	Bacilli are sensitive to antileprosy drugs
8. Resistance of *M. leprae* to the drugs can be demonstrated on culture in the foot pad of thymectomized, irradiated or nude mice	-
Alternative drugs (Ethionamide/Prothionamide) may be added	Restart MDT

Table 20.3: Criteria differentiating relapse from type 1 (Lepra) reaction

Relapse	Type 1 (Lepra) Reaction
1. Adequately treated as per WHO recommendations	May or may not have received adequate treatment
2. Complete subsidence of disease with no residual clinical or histopathological evidence of activity	Disease may not have subsided completely
3. Reappearance of lesions from a few previously involved areas or a part of the area involved by previous lesions	Appearance of lesions at fresh, previously clinically normal sites
4. Classification remains constant	Upgrading BT←BB←BL, Downgrading BT→BB→BL
5. Reappearance of nerve involvement in nerves which had become quiescent following adequate treatment	Fresh nerve involvement in addition to aggravation of previously involved nerves
6. Reappearance of activity is insidious and may occur long after treatment is stopped	Onset is usually acute and severe
7. Histopathology and lepromin reaction conform to classification of the previous episode	There is change in histopathological and lepromin findings during the reactional episode
Responds to multidrug therapy (MDT) alone.	Treatment of reaction required in addition to MDT
No apparent systemic signs or symptoms	May be accompanied by constitutional signs and symptoms

RECOMMENDED READING

1. Baker RJ. The need for new drugs in the treatment and control of leprosy. *Int J Lepr Other Mycobact Dis*. 1990;58:78-97.
2. Chopra NK, Aggarwal JS, Pandya PG. A study of relapse in paucibacillary leprosy in a multidrug therapy project, Baroda District, India. *Lepr Rev*. 1990;61:157-162.
3. Jacobson RR, Hastings RC. Rifampin-resistant leprosy. *Lancet*. 1976;2:1304-1305.
4. Ji BH. Anonymous. Expert committee on leprosy. Sixth Technical Report Series NO. 768, WHO, Geneva 14, 1988.
5. Ji BH. Drug resistance in leprosy—a review. *Lepr Rev*. 1985;56:265-278.
6. Katoch K, Ramanathan V, Natarajan M, Bagga AK, Bhatia AS, Saxena RK, et al. Relapse in paucibacillary patients after treatment with three short-term regimens containing rifampin. *Int J Lepr Other Mycobact Dis*. 1989;57:458-464.
7. Meade TW, Pearson JMH, Rees RJW, North WRS. The epidemiology of sulfone-resistant leprosy. *Int J Lepr*, 1973;41:684.
8. Pearson JM, Haile GS, Barnetson RS, Rees RJ. Dapsone resistant leprosy in Ethiopia. *Lepr Rev*. 1979;50:183-199.
9. Pearson JM, Rees RJ, Waters MF. Sulfone resistance in leprosy. A review of one hundred proven clinical cases. *Lancet*. 1975;2:69-72.
10. Pettit JH, Rees RJ, Ridley DS. Studies on sulfone resistance in leprosy I. Detection of cases. *Int J Lepr Other Mycobact Dis*. 1966;34:375-390.
11. Rees RJ, Waters MF, Pearson JM, Helmy HS, Laing AB. Long-term treatment of dapsone-resistant leprosy with refampicin; clinical and bacteriological studies. *Int J Lepr Other Mycobact Dis*. 1976;44:159-169.
12. Sehgal VN, Bhattacharya SN, Jain S. Relapse or late reversal reaction? *Int J Lepr Other Mycobact Dis*. 1990;58:118-121.
13. Sehgal VN, Joginder. Slit-skin smear in leprosy. *Int J Dermatol*. 1990;29:9-16.
14. Taylor PM, Chacko CJG, Job CK. Study of sulfone resistance in leprosy patients in India. *Int J Lepr*. 1982;50:123-127.
15. Waters MF, Rees RJ, McDougall AC, Weddell AG. Ten years of dapsone in lepromatous leprosy: clinical, bacteriological and histological assessment and the findings of viable leprosy bacilli. *Lepr Rev*. 1974;45:288-298.

Urban Leprosy

Urban leprosy is indeed intriguing entity for its increasing impact on leprosy control. It has emerged as a definitive entity in the recent past. It is, therefore, imperative to define the entity. Urban leprosy incorporates known leprosy patients or those identified through their cardinal presenting features or referred by other doctors, and those detected accidentally when they report for other ailments at urban leprosy centers irrespective of their place of residence. It also includes leprosy patients detected through surveys in the urban areas. The latter have received scant attention so far.

EPIDEMIOLOGY

The clinical picture of urban leprosy is now clearly defined. It affects largely persons of a younger age group: 20–29 years though no age group is immune. Males are affected more frequently than females. Similarly, the common age at onset is 29 years. Unskilled workers and those coming from low socioeconomic strata are common among them. Urban leprosy *per se* is not a major problem, but transmigration of population from endemic belts due primarily to economic reasons magnifies the problem. Thus, urbanization plays an important part in the emergence of urban leprosy. The most startling finding of urban leprosy is that the large majority of patients are of the infectious type comprising borderline-tuberculoid, mid-borderline, borderline-lepromatous and lepromatous, a pattern quite different for that in endemic belts. Keeping in

view the findings on urban leprosy, a further activity should be initiated to define the quantum of the urban leprosy problem so that stringent measures to check such a situation may be taken.

PREVENTIVE MEASURES

It is suggested that the following measures be undertaken for preventing the problem from taking enlarged dimensions.

Creation of awareness: It is very crucial to create awareness about leprosy in the minds of the general public and doctors. This can be achieved by widespread coverage of leprosy in newspapers, radio, television and other information media.

Undergraduate and postgraduate training: It is vital to include the teaching of leprosy in the undergraduate curriculum so as to expose the students to the magnitude of the problem in the country. Atleast 15 days out of rotating internship should be devoted to leprosy training. It would also be desirable to have a postgraduate qualification exclusively in this subject, namely a diploma (D Lep) or MD degree in leprosy.

Training of paramedical personnel: Adequate number of paramedical personnel should be trained to identify and treat leprosy cases.

Uniform applicability of National Leprosy Eradication Program: On account of rapid migration of people from one place to another, it is proposed that no area in a country should be considered free from leprosy and the program should be uniformly enforced in endemic as well as in so called non-endemic areas.

Uniform pattern of leprosy: It is imperative to form a consensus regarding the therapy of leprosy. Multidrug therapy should form the main stay in infectious leprosy in order to (a) render the cases noninfectious as early as possible and (b) to prevent the emergence of dapsone resistance. The treatment should be specific, adequate and regular.

Creation of health check-posts: It is important to create health check-posts for identifying the infectious cases at railway stations, airport, interstate bus stands and at the borders of the states. This will assist in the detection of infectious cases at the point of entry to city. It is at that point only that these patients should be issued an identify card mentioning the type of leprosy and details of treatment, with the advice to report to a particular urban leprosy center so that he should be brought under treatment at the earlier possible time, besides, he should be properly informed about the nature of this particular disease, its repercussions on the family members and the society in general.

Physical and economic rehabilitation: All those patients who have been treated and are under surveillance should be rehabilitated both physically and economically to ensure that they become self-sufficient. However, those patients who are on treatment for a requisite period should also be considered for restoration to suitable jobs on the basis of an assessment in each individual case.

A change from urbanization to ruralization: It is high time that the health authorities in consultation with the other relevant bodies should enforce a change from urbanization to ruralization. This envisages setting up of industries in the villages in order to provide job incentives to the rural population so that present day trend of transmigration from rural to the checking the influx of leprosy patients in cities. Furthermore, institution of specialized facilities for leprosy treatment in the rural areas may impede their search better medical facilities in big cities.

Population surveys: Urban surveys should be undertaken and these should have the components of surveys in urban slums, school surveys and surveys of industrial areas. Hospital surveys should also be utilized to evaluate the problem of urban leprosy.

Legal measures: The prevailing legal measures in different countries amount to discrimination against leprosy patients. They should, therefore, be liberalized. The word leper should be eliminated while adopting new measures. Control of leprosy should form a part of other infectious diseases control. Accordingly, the measures adopted for their control should also be applicable to leprosy. It should be worthwhile to combine the facilities for the examination of leprosy patients and their contacts, defining them as infectious or noninfectious. Further measures should include notification of infectious cases in particular and noninfectious in general, administration of specific, adequate and regular treatment and the creation of facilities to treat infectious and acutely ill patients in institutions. Preparation or sale of food, drinks, drugs or clothing taking drinking water or bathing or washing clothes in public wells and tanks by infectious cases should be restricted as far as possible. The implication of such restrictions should also be explained to them so that they would not feel offended.

▌RECOMMENDED READING

1. Sehgal VN, Ghorpade A, Saha K, Urban leprosy-an appraisal from northern India. *Lep Rev.* 1984;55:159-166.

Prevention and Control of Leprosy

Leprosy is one of the major public health problems all over the globe. In spite of endeavors by the international agencies, leprosy controls has not been as successful as in other communicable disease. It is largely because the *Mycobacterium leprae* has thus far defied the researchers, and even the Koch's postulates have remained unfulfilled. In order, to assess the magnitude of leprosy and check its perpetuation and spread, active participation of medical, paramedical personnel, community, voluntary agencies and the government authority is essential and of course, the leprosy patient is the pivot in the control of the disease.

Assessment of the Magnitude

It is essential to make an assessment of the leprosy control in an area, state or the country. This forms the basis for creation of facilities, which may vary from country to country.

The ideal leprosy control program should comprise control centers at the rural, district and state levels with a central directing authority. These centers have to carry out the functions of case findings, treatment, rehabilitation, social welfare and health education.

Case Finding

Different methods are employed for case findings, the easiest being the examination of contacts of known leprosy patients. The same is enlarged to find the contacts. The other methods are group surveys-school, industries, mills, factories, camps- and/or house to house census surveys.

TREATMENT

All the patients must be brought under the network of the center for treatment. Adequate, specific and regular treatment should be ensured. Maintenance of treatment records is obligatory as it helps in follow-up and tracing the defaulters. Domiciliary treatment may be introduced, especially for defaulters.

Side by side the patient should be explained the advantages of treatment of leprosy and its effect on control and progress of the disease. Furthermore, it is imperative to create facilities for indoor treatment of acute complications of the disease. In addition, facilities for dressing of ulcers and physiotherapy for preventing deformities should be made available. Similarly, referral centers may be created for specialized treatment where complications and deformities can also be effectively managed.

Social Welfare and Rehabilitation

The rehabilitation of the patient should start from the day of his diagnosis. Physiological rehabilitation of the patient is vital; sympathetic attitude and understanding of the patient is of considerable assistance. It helps in gaining the confidence of the patient and changing his attitude towards leprosy. Early preventive measures to minimize the deformities should be adopted—physiotherapy surgery forms an important link in rehabilitation of the patient.

The leprosy workers should help in finding suitable jobs for the patients so that they become self-sufficient and useful for the society. Financial assistance through welfare agencies would also be useful to them.

Health Education

It is achieved by educating the patient, the public health workers, administrators and politicians.

Patients' education: It is aimed at infusing hope, gaining confidence and to encourage them to take regular treatment. Special instructions should be given to them to take care of the anesthetic hands, feet and eyes to prevent ulcers and deformities. Infectious patients in particular are educated to avoid skin to skin contact with others, live separately, avoid marriage, hence helping in controlling the disease. They may be encouraged to get sterilized.

Public education: The objectives should be to explain to the public, the nature of the disease in order to rout out the prejudices, and to encourage a rational attitude towards the disease and the persons suffering from it. They should be educated to seek medical opinion on suspicion of leprosy and to notify the known cases to the authorities.

Education of health workers: The health personnel concerned with leprosy control program such as doctors, paramedical staff and medical social workers, should be imparted training to deal effectively with the disease. The details of pattern of training have to be worked out to suit the actual requirements of the individual countries or areas. This envisages the criteria for their selection, the contents of the course and its duration. Time to time evaluation of the efficacy of teaching and learning methods should be undertaken. It is imperative to complement the training program with refresher courses. The teaching of leprosy should form an essential content of the undergraduate curriculum in medical colleges, in order to bring much mooted integration of leprosy in the health services. General practitioners should be trained to change their attitude towards leprosy and treat the leprosy patients in the same way as other patients. In addition, it is incumbent on them to educate the public in this direction as discussed above.

Education of administrators and politicians: Similarly, the attitude of the administrators. Politicians, policy planners need to be changed by apprising them about the magnitude of the leprosy problem and its aftermath. This may ensured the adequate allocation of funds required to execute the planning and control of leprosy.

Implementation of Program

In order to carry out the aforesaid activities, adequate administrative set up is essential, which may differ from country to country. In India at present, the pattern of leprosy control as practiced is described here.

Leprosy control units: They are located in rural areas having moderate to high prevalence rate (0.5 percent and above). Each unit consists of full time trained medical officer, and a number of non-medical supervisors, and paramedical personnel.

Survey, education and training (SET) centers: This consists of a paramedical worker who is responsible for conducting the above mentioned activities. He works under the supervision of the medical officer of the primary health center or the dispensary. Many such SET centers, depending upon the population covered, may be attached to a primary health center.

Urban leprosy center: It is located in an urban area and is attached to a hospital. Only a senior paramedical worker carries out health education and survey of certain groups under the guidance of the medical officer in charge.

Leprosy referral center: Medical colleges and other suitable institutions where consultative facilities are available for leprosy are made use of in control program. These centers are called referral centers.

Temporary hospitalization of acutely ill patients: New facilities are being created or existing facilities are being utilized for indoor treatment of acutely ill patients in the medical college, hospitals, district hospitals or leprosy homes as a part of leprosy control program.

Administrative set-up: The above mentioned centers are located at different levels. They work under the direction of the respective state directorate of health services. They in turn are being guided by the director general of health services who is responsible for supervising the national leprosy eradication program.

Segregation

It forms a salient link in the control and spread of leprosy. The isolation of infectious cases is best achieved by indoor treatment. The creation of leprosoria is ideal. However, in view of lack of financial resources, it is beyond the reach of developing countries. Hence, the meager indoor facilities should be judiciously used for infectious patients, especially from households where higher incidence is noted. Improvised method to reduce exposure may be used according to the need of the individual such as isolation in the house, avoidance of skin contact and the like.

Chemoprophylaxis

Its value has not yet been established. It may, however, be used especially in children who are in close contact with infectious cases. Dapsone is used for the purpose in convenient dosage as described in the 'therapy of leprosy'. The prophylactic treatment should continue till the index case becomes non-infective or till the contacts are separated.

BCG Prophylaxis

Use of BCG in prophylaxis of leprosy is still debatable. The BCG vaccination sometimes converts a lepromin negative reaction into a positive one. It is in these patients, BCG may be of help in providing protection against *Mycobacterium leprae*, especially in children upto the age of five years.

23

Chemotherapy

Multidrug therapy (MDT), recommended for the first time, had the salient chief characteristics namely:

- The regimens were comprised of several drugs acting by different mechanisms, in order to prevent the emergence of drug resistance, and also effective against the dapsone resistant strains of *Mycobacterium leprae*:
- The duration of the regimens was limited, in contrast to the life long duration of dapsone monotherapy, to ensure patients' compliance. Accordingly, only bactericidal drugs were included for the purpose:
- Rifampicin (RMP) forms its key component, because of its powerful bactericidal effect against *M. leprae*. It was required to be administered under supervision only once a month to insure compliance and because of its high cost;
- The recommended regimens were the minimal effective regimens; there was no recommendation against the use of stronger/longer regimens.

▌OFFICIAL REGIMENS

Three regimens have officially been recommended;
- WHO/MDT for paucibacillary (PB) leprosy;
- WHO/MDT for multibacillary (MB) leprosy; and
- A single dose containing RMP-ofloxacin-minocycline (ROM) for single-lesion PB leprosy. The later is to be employed in the countries,

where the proportion of single lesion PB patients is large.

The composition of the two-regimens, which were recommended by a WHO study group, has so far remained unchanged. However, the definitions of PB and MB leprosy have been modified on several occasions, and the cut-off point between PB and MB leprosy has been simplified from a bacterial index (BI) of $\geq$ 2 + in the initial skin smears at any site to more than five skin lesions. Consequently, a larger proportion of newly detected patients are classified as MB leprosy as compared to those in the past. Simultaneously, the duration of MDT for MB leprosy has gradually been shortened, from 'at least 2 years, and, whenever possible, until skin smears negativity, to a total of 24 months. At its seventh meeting, the WHO Expert Committee on Leprosy stated that 24-month duration for MB leprosy remained valid, while suggesting that 'it is possible that the duration of the current MDT regimen for multibacillary leprosy could be further shortened to 12 months. This careful wording clearly indicates that the recommended duration of MDT for MB leprosy is either 24 or 12 months.

The third regimen, a single dose of ROM for the treatment of single-lesion PB leprosy, which possesses obvious operational advantages, was also recommended as an alternative, has subsequently been applied widely in Indian subcontinent, Bangladesh and Brazil.

NEW MDT REGIMENS

The need for new regimens that are more effective operationally and less demanding are being outlined:
- From the operational point of view, the recommended duration of treatment, particularly for MB leprosy, is still too long;
- Two of the components of the current regimen for MB leprosy—dapsone and clofazimine—are only weakly bactericidal against the organism, since it is these drugs that determine the minimal effective duration of the current regimen, further shortening of its duration might result in higher relapse rates;
- Administration of the daily components, dapsone and clofazimine, are hard to supervise, as a result of which the MDT regimen for MB leprosy is not 'resistance-proof', should patients fail to comply with treatment;
- Patients who do not tolerate clofazimine either because of skin pigmentation, or dapsone or RMP hypersensitivity, or unable to benefit from RMP due to intercurrent disease or the emergence of RMP resistance strains of *M. leprae*, require a safe and effective alternative.

The discovery of new drugs that demonstrate very promising bactericidal activity against *M. leprae* has made possible the formulation of new MDT regimens. A highly desirable new regimen is one that would permit all of the components to be administered once monthly under supervision, significantly reducing the risk of emergence of RMP resistance caused by irregular administration of the daily components. ROM is the first fully supervisable, monthly-administered regimen. The efficacy of multiple monthly doses of ROM for treatment of MB and PB leprosy has been tested in field trials. Furthermore, because of the success of a single dose of ROM for the treatment of single-lesion PB leprosy, the treatment of multiple-lesion PB leprosy with a single dose of ROM should be evaluated. Should this treatment be successful, the chemotherapy of PB leprosy could be much simplified, saving significant resources that may be used for other important activities.

The bactericidal activities of both ofloxacin and minocycline are rather weak, compared with that of RMP; the combination ofloxacin-minocycline is significantly less active than is RMP alone, and ROM is no more bactericidal than is RMP alone. Replacing the components of ROM with more powerfully bactericidal drugs would make possible a fully supervisible, monthly-administered MDT regimen. Recent findings from experiments in mice indicate that rifapentine and moxifloxacin are significantly more bactericidal than are RMP and ofloxacin, respectively, and the combination refapentine—moxifloxacin-minocycline (PMM) is far more bactericidal than ROM. The efficacy of PMM is currently being measured in a short-term clinical trial among lepromatous leprosy patients. If the trial confirms the stronger bactericidal effect of PMM, a field trial to evaluate the efficacy and side-effects of PMM over the long-term should be carried out.

A common regimen for the treatment of both PB and MB leprosy is desirable. However, because PB and MB leprosy differ so greatly in terms of the size of the bacterial population and the underlying immunological response, the requirements for chemotherapy, especially in terms of the number of drugs and the basis of the available drugs, It appears likely that it would over treat PB or under treat MB. The dream of a common regimen might be realized only if the new regimen contained several very powerful bactericidal drugs, which are capable of shortening the duration of treatment for MB leprosy to only few doses or even to a single dose.

Recently, the WHO Technical Advisory Group (TAG), at its third meeting, recommended that all leprosy patients, both PB and MB, be treated by the MDT regimen for MB leprosy for a period of only 6 months. The TAG stated, in support of this recommendation, that:
- MDT has been proven to be robust in terms of treatment, efficacy and safety;
- Relapse rates are very low, less than 1 percent; and
- Resistance to MDT has been virtually non-existent.

However, that regimen is effective and safe is not sufficient to justify shortening of its duration.

A good example is THELEP regimen C, which was composed of a single dose of RMP plus daily dapsone administered for a period of 2 years; this regimen was highly effective and safe, but 20 percent of the patients allocated to this regimen relapsed after an average of 5 years of follow-up. Since 1998, almost all MB patients have been treated with 12 months MDT; however, no information is available regarding the 5-year relapse rate following 12 months MDT. Therefore, at least for the time being, there is no justification for further shortening of the duration of MB chemotherapy to 6 months. Moreover, it appears hazardous to state that resistance does not exist, because post-MDT surveillance has not been carried out in routine programs for almost 10 years. For these reasons, before any proposal to shorten further duration of treatment for MB leprosy by the current MDT regimen or of a common regimen for both PB and MB leprosy may be implemented in control programs, these proposals must be studies by controlled trials, with relapse at the outcome.

Magnitudes of MB relapse after multidrug therapy (MDT) and possible existence of a higher risk subgroup of multibacillary (MB) leprosy.

Among MB patients, the efficacy of MDT is best assessed by measuring the relapse rate after completion of treatment. The relapse rate was reported to be about 0–1 percent per annum among MB patients administered MDT for 24 months. Because of the low relapse rates, post-MDT surveillance has been discontinued. However, reports from the Institute Marchoux in Bamako and the Central JALMA Institute in Agra indicate the existence of a subgroup of MB patients who demonstrate a high frequency of relapse after 24-month MDT, as high as 4–7 per 100 patient-years among patients with initial mean BI $\geq$ 4.0, and far higher than that among patients with initial BI < 4.0, suggesting that the high initial BI is a most important risk factor for relapse. In addition, relapse was observed to occur late, 5 years after stopping treatment, on an average, suggesting that follow-up of these patients may be important. Because there is no ready explanation of the discrepancy between the two estimates of the risk of the relapse among MB patients after 24 months MDT, and the possible existence of a subgroup of MB patients who are more prone to relapse, it is necessary to collect more information from the long-term follow-up of MB patients after completion of 24 months MDT. However, a number of difficulties are encountered in attempting to follow former MB patients after completion of MDT:

- In more and more routine programs, the patients are removed from the register as soon as they have completed MDT, and very often, essential records, like identity, address, initial BI and history of treatment, are lost, making it difficult to retrieve patients for follow-up and analysis;
- Because of integration of the leprosy program into the general health services, responsibility for the detection of suspected relapse rests upon general health workers, many of whom do not possess the necessary skills. In addition, the general health services often lack the manpower and resources required to follow former patients who have already completed their treatment with MDT, because they are no longer considered 'cases; and
- Because of the poor quality of skin smears in the past, and because a skin smear service is no longer available in many programs, it is difficult to identify members of the higher-risk subgroup and to detect relapse.

Because no information exists with respect to the 5-year relapse rate among MB patients after 12 months MDT, determination of the relapse rate following 12-month MDT should be considered a high priority in those treatment centers in which post-treatment surveillance is possible. In addition, the results of ongoing trials, in which the relapse rates after treatment by various regimens, including the 12-month regimen, are compared, should be published as soon as they become available.

NEEDS FOR BOTH FLEXIBILITY AND RELIABILITY OF MDT TREATMENT

To guarantee that all newly detected leprosy patients receive treatment with MDT, the MDT services should be available and accessible to the patients. To accomplish this goal, flexible, patient-friendly system for delivery of MDT must be implemented.

However, at the same time, the principle that monthly RMP is to be administered under supervision should not be compromised, because RMP is the single, most important component of MDT, and non-compliance of leprosy patients with treatment have been well documented. In addition, the importance of regular contact between patient and health worker for the purpose of preventing of impairment must not be underestimated.

In areas in which the infrastructure is weak, there are patients who may find it difficult to visit the health center once monthly. Currently policy states that 'in such cases, more than a months' supply of MDT blister-packs may be provided to the patient, and that with 'accompanied MDT', blister-packs for a full course of MDT should be provided at the time of diagnosis. Constantly, in an increasing number of national programs, it has become the routine to provide the entire quantity of MDT blister-packs—6-month supply for PB and a 12-month supply for MB patients—to all newly detected patients. However, in many programs, those responsible for 'accompanying' the patients' treatment either have not been recruited, or lack proper training, as a result of which many of them fail to carry out their mission. As a consequence, it is difficult to be certain that the MDT drugs are indeed self-administers by the patients, notwithstanding the fact that the success of MDT could be seriously jeopardized, should patients be non-compliant.

Because the monthly component was expected to be administered under supervision, studies of compliance with MDT undertaken since the introduction of MDT focused on regularity of self-administration of the daily component, chiefly dapsone, by urine testing. Whereas the results demonstrated better compliance with MDT than with dapsone monotherapy, only 70–80 percent of patients were found in compliance with the daily component, suggesting that the assumption that 'patients who report for diagnosis and treatment may be considered as sufficiently motivated to take full responsibility for their own care, may not be valid. Although one of the advantages of the blister-pack over the supply of MDT drugs in bulk was assumed to be improved patient compliance with the self-administered component, this assumption

has been tested in only a few studies; these studies have demonstrated that blister-packs either did not improve compliance, or improved it only, marginally.

Because the monthly component is no longer administered under supervision to a significant proportion of patients, it appears very likely that reduction of the frequency of contact between patients and health workers will affect the regularity of drug administration; therefore, compliance with both the monthly and daily components of MDT is certainly an issue far more important and complicated than before. It is important to measure the degree of non-compliance among those who are treated under the policy of flexible drug delivery with both the daily and the monthly components of the MDT blister pack. This may have significant impact on MDT delivery policy, and even on the strategy of the chemotherapy of leprosy.

'Accompanied MDT' is the term applied to a program in which a family or a community member supervises the monthly administration of drugs to the patient. This concept appears reasonable, but before its wide implementation, this approach should be tested under field condition, to identify the requirements for its success. However, even with the best program of 'accompanied MDT', the justification for providing the total quantity of MDT drugs to the patient may be disputed, because the family or community member cannot replace the health worker.

ABSENTEEISM AND DEFAULT

A defaulter has been defined as a patient who has not collected MDT treatment for 12 consecutive months, and that the register is updated at least annually. In number of national programs, 40 percent of newly detected patients have been considered defaulters. Since introduction of the 'flexible MDT delivery' strategy, increasing numbers of patients have received the entire quantity of MDT drugs at the time of the first dose of treatment. Although it has stated that the percentage of defaulters has declined dramatically as a result of this approach, it is difficult to assess the actual rate of completion of treatment.

Whatever the reason for default, every effort should be made to prevent it. A serious attempt should be made to trace absentees beginning at the time of their first absence. Absentees who return to treatment should be treated according to WHO recommendations: six doses of MDT within 9 months for PB; and 12 doses within 18 months for MB. In addition, tracing and persuading the defaulters to return for treatment is most important.

For those patients who have become defaulters, those who have died or migrated from the country should be removed from the register, whereas those who have moved out of the district or are taking treatment elsewhere should be transferred rather than simply removed from register. As long as the defaulters continue to live in the district and have yet to complete the full course of MDT treatment, they remain, by definition, 'cases', and may continue to represent sources of transmission. Instead of removing these defaulters from the register, health workers should be encouraged to retrieve them actively, with assistance from the community. A few courses of MDT should be given to every defaulter after his retrieval or return.

DRUG RESISTANCE

To date, all of the official MDT regimens contain RMP, which is significantly more bactericidal than any other antileprosy drug or any combination of ofloxacin, clarithromycin and minocycline. Emergence of RMP resistance would pose a serious threat to the achievement of leprosy control.

Rifampicin (RMP) resistant leprosy was first documented in the 1970s. It was rare, probably because, in that era, RMP was seldom employed for the treatment of leprosy. Later, it was reported that, among a total of 404 MB patients who had been treated with various RMP-containing regimens, 39 relapsed and 22 were found to harbour organisms resistant to RMP, as proven by the mouse footpad technique. Virtually all of the resistant strains were isolated from patients who had been treated with RMP only after they had relapsed after long-term monotherapy with dapsone or other sulfones, and almost all of the strains were also resistant to dapsone, indicating that these patients had in effect been receiving RMP monotherapy. Because many

of the 22 patients developed RMP resistance in the decade after beginning treatment with RMP, it appeared that RMP resistance could emerge rather rapidly among patients whose treatment regimens were inappropriate.

Although more than 10 million leprosy patients in the world have completed treatment with MDT, and RMP resistant leprosy has not been reported among these patients, one must be cautions in interpreting the findings.

Post-MDT surveillance for relapse is no longer carried out in most routine programs.

The standard means of diagnosing drug resistant leprosy has required use of the mouse footpad techniques, however, the great majority of the mouse footpad laboratories established for surveys of dapsone resistance have disappeared during the last decade, which coincided with intensive implementation of MDT.

As a result, RMP-susceptibility testing is rarely carried out, and the results are not always reliable. In fact, one cannot exclude the possibility that a number of RMP resistant leprosy patients are currently undetected. Before RMP resistance becomes so frequent that it threatens leprosy control, more solid information about its magnitude should be collected in different parts of the world.

Although, it is no longer feasible to undertake a relatively large-scale survey of RMP resistant leprosy through mouse footpad technique yet, PCR-based DNA sequence analysis of the *rpoB* gene of *M. leprae* represents a cost-effective alternative technique. At this stage, surveys of RMP resistance should focus on MB patients who have relapsed after completion of MDT, and surveillance for the emergence of RMP resistance among relapsed MB patients should be carried out by special centers, for this purpose, a proportion of MB patients should be systematically examined clinically and bacteriologically after completion of MDT, and skin biopsy specimens should be obtained from those patients suspected of relapse for DNA sequence analysis of the *rpoB* gene of *M. leprae*.

Multidrug therapy (MDT) was developed mainly because of the widespread emergence of dapsone resistance, and the MDT regimens were designed on the principle that they would be effective against all the strains of *M. leprae* regardless of their susceptibility to dapsone. Hence, in the MDT era, whether the global prevalence of dapsone resistance is increasing or declining is virtually irrelevant to the therapeutic effect of MDT, and there is no need to monitor trends of resistance to dapsone.

RECOMMENDATION

- To guarantee the quality of leprosy services, training in leprosy should be strengthened among general health workers.
- The skin smear remains an important tool for diagnosing MB relapse; wherever possible, it should be reintroduced, particularly in areas in which there are a significant number of MB patients who have completed MDT, or the prevalence is greater than 1 per 10,000 population.
- Currently, almost all MB patients are being treated by 12-month MDT, however, no information is available regarding the 5-year relapse rate among MB patients treated by this regimen. Therefore,

field programs with adequate facilities should monitor the relapse rates, surveillance among relapsed MB patients for the emergence of rifampicin resistance should be carried out by special centers.

- A flexible, patient-friendly system for delivery of MDT must be implemented. At the same time, the principle that monthly RMP is to be administered under supercision should not be compromised. Only in exceptional cases, in which the patients cannot be seen monthly, should more than a 1-month supply of MDT blister packs be provided.
- Health workers should actively trace absentees and encourage them to complete their treatment, instead of passively awaiting their return and removing them as defaulter from the register after an absence of 12 or more consecutive months.

The preceding predicaments of the current therapy may successfully be surmounted by the current recommendation of modified therapy (Table 23.1).

Table 23.1: Current recommendation for chemotherapy

Clinical group	Drugs	Dose	Mode of administration	Duration
Paucibacillary I, TT, BT (PB)	Rifampicin	600 mg	Once a month, supervised	6 doses in 9 months (maximum gap: 8 weeks)
Dapsone Toxicity	Dapsone Clofazimine	100 mg 50 mg	Daily, self-administered Daily, self-administered (in lieu of dapsone)	6 months (maximum gap: 4 weeks) 6 months (maximum gap: 4 weeks)
Multibacillary BT (MB), BB, BL, LL	Rifampicin	600 mg	Once a month, supervised	24 doses in 36 months (No single gap > 8 weeks)
	Clofazimine	300 mg	Once a month, supervised	24 doses in 36 months (No single gap > 8 weeks)
		50 mg	Daily, self-administered	24 monthly cycles in 36 months (no gap > 4 weeks)
	Dapsone	100 mg	Daily, self-administered	24 monthly cycles in 36 months (no gap > 4 weeks)
Relapse/Rifampicin Resistance/Toxicity	Clofazimine	50 mg	Daily, self-administered Plus 2 out of 3 daily (in lieu of dapsone)	6 months followed by
	Ofloxacin (1) Minocycline (2)	400 mg	(Clofazimine plus ofloxacin or minocycline daily)	18 months Total 24 monthly cycles in 36 months (no gap > 4 weeks)
	Clarithromycin (3)	250 mg		

[*Courtesy:* Bhattacharya SN, Sehgal VN. An reappraisal of drifting scenario of Leprosy multi-drug therapy (MDT): a proposal for fresh approach in the new millennium. Int J Dermatol. 2002;41:321-326.]

■ RECOMMENDED READING

1. Anonymous. WHO expert Committee on Leprosy. Seventh Report. WHO Technical Report Series no. 874, World Health Organization, 1998, Geneva.

2. Anonymous. WHO Study Group. Chemotherapy of Leprosy. WHO Technical Report Series no. 847. World Health Organization, 1994, Geneva.

3. Anonymous. WHO study group. Chemotherapy of leprosy for control programmes. WHO technical Report Series no. 675. World Health Organization, 1982, Geneva.

4. Bhattacharya SN, Sehgal VN. An reappraisal of drifting scenario of Leprosy multidrug therapy: new approach proposal for fresh approach in the new millennium. *Int J Dermatol*. 2002;41:321-326.

5. Bhattacharya SN, Sehgal VN. Leprosy elimination campaign and its impending fallouts. *Int J Dermatol*. 2000;39:667-669.

6. Cambau E, Bonnafous P, Perani E, Sougakoff W, Ji B, Jarlier V. Molecular detection of rifampin and ofloxacin resistance for patients who experienced relapse of multibacillary leprosy. *Clin Infect Dis*, 2002;34:39-45.

7. Consigny S, Bentoucha A, Bonnafous P, Grosset J, Ji B. Bactericidal activities of HMR 3647, moxifloxacin, and refapentine against *Mycobacterium leprae* in mice. *Antimicrob Agents Chemother*. 2000;44:2919-2921.

8. Daumeric D. Current World Health Organization-sponsored studies in the chemotherapy of leprosy. *Lepr Rev*. 2000;71:S88-90.

9. Honore N, Cole ST. Molecular basis of rifampin resistance in *Mycobacterium leprae*. *Antimicrob Agents Chemother*. 1993;37:414-418.

10. Honore N, Perani E, Telenti A, Grosset J, Cole ST. A simple and rapid technique for the detection of rifampin resistance in *Mycobacterium leprae*. *Int J Lepr Other Mycobact Dis*. 1993;61:600-604.

11. Ji B, Sow S, Perani E, Lienhardt C, Diderot V, Grosset J. Bactericidal activity of a single dose combination of ofloxacin plus minocycline, with or without rifampin, against *Mycobacterium leprae* in mice and in lepromatous patients. *Antimicrob Agents Chemother*. 1998;42:1115-1120.

12. Ji B. Prospect for chemotherapy of leprosy. *Indian J Lepr*. 2000;72:35-46.

13. Sehgal VN, Sardana K, Dogra S. Management of complications following leprosy: an evolving scenario. *J Dermatolog Treat*. 2007;18:366-374.

14. Sehgal VN, Sardana K, Dogra S. The imperatives of leprosy treatment in the pre- and post-global leprosy elimination era: appraisal of changing the scenario to current status. *J Dermatolog Treat*. 2008;19:82-91.

15. Shepard CC. A brief review of experience with short-term clinical trials monitored by mouse foot pad inoculation. *Lepr Rev*. 1981;52:299-308.

24   Epidemiology and Control

Leprosy elimination was defined in 1991 as prevalence smaller than one per 10,000 inhabitants. Underlying the elimination strategy was the hypothesis that, because leprosy patients are assumed to be the sole source of infection, early detection and treatment of the cases by MDT would reduce transmission of the organism. Once the prevalence fell down a certain level, incidence would be reduced; in the long-term, the chain transmission would be broken, and leprosy would disappear naturally.

It is now necessary to seek evidence to verify this hypotheses. Some important questions must be answered concerning the effectiveness of interventions to reduce transmission of *M. leprae* and the sources of infection. Evidence concerning these issues will be reviewed here. The validity of several indicators for leprosy epidemiology and control will also be discussed.

Are untreated MB patients the only significant source of infection?

Untreated MB patients are most probably the most important source of transmission of *M. leprae*. Houshold contacts of multibacillary patients have been estimated to have a risk of developing leprosy 5–10 times greater than that of the general population, and a positive association exists between smear positivity and infectiousness. In low endemic situations, relative risk associated with household contact could even be greater.

Several studies have shown that untreated MB patients excrete quantities of *M. leprae* from

the nose and mouth. However, many studies have suggested that untreated MB patients do not represent the sole source of infection. Household contacts of paucibacillary (PB) patients have also been shown to be at greater risk of developing the disease than are non-contacts, although the risk is smaller than that to contacts of MB patients. It is possible that the PB patients are not themselves the source of transmission; rather, the household contact has had contact with some outside source of infection. Those who join the household of an MB patient after treatment has been started have been shown to be at lower risk than the contacts of untreated MB cases, but at greater risk than the general population. If MDT renders the index case noninfectious, it appears likely that the source of infection is not the index case directly, but the environment of the household.

Because, in many areas, the numbers of MB patients are very small, they may not represent the most important source of infection. There is increasing evidence that sub clinical transmission may occur. Nasal excretion of *M. leprae* by subclinically infected individuals could be responsible for transmission, although this is not proven. DNA sequence apparently unique to *M. leprae* have been isolated on nasal swabs from many apparently healthy individuals residing in endemic areas and large proportions of those who live in areas endemic for leprosy have been shown to demonstrate seropositivity against *M. leprae* specific antigens. Even in highly endemic countries, no history of close contact with a leprosy patient can be established for many patients, although a study carried out in one endemic village in Indonesia showed that some contact with a leprosy patient could be demonstrated for most incident cases.

Direct spread is certainly important, but infection may also be indirect. *M. leprae*, which have been said to be capable of survival outside the human body for as long as several months under favorable conditions, have also been found in the soil. Insect bites have also been said to be capable of transmitting the organism. This latter route of infection is probably not very efficient, but it cannot be completely dismissed as a possibility. The existence of extra-human, animal reservoirs of *M. leprae-* specific DNA has been reported to be present in water, and the risk of leprosy was to be correlated with the use of contaminated water for bathing and washing. Leprosy lesions following dog-bites, vaccinations and tattoing have also been reported. Nude mice, the feet of which had been smeared with *M. leprae* and also pricked with contaminated thorns, developed leprosy lesions, and infection of wild armadillos through thorn pricks has also been suspected; such a route of infection cannot be completely excluded for humans. Finally, in some settings, the anatomical distribution of the lesions in patients with a single macule strongly suggests transcutaneous infection through wounds. Other studies of the anatomical distribution of lesions are not consistent with this hypothesis, but could be consistent with infections through insect-bites.

What evidence is there for the effectiveness of interventions to stop or reduce the incidence of leprosy?

IMPACT OF MDT ON TRANSMISSION

MDT greatly reduces the infectiousness of leprosy patients in a matter of a few days, a period of time such shorter than that required by dapsone monotherapy (approximately 3 months). Although incidence rates have been observed to have declined in many settings, evidence that MDT caused an acceleration

of that decline is rare. In many places, the decline of incidence began before the introduction of MDT, or could be explained as well by other factors. In other settings, no decline of incidence has been observed, despite the routine administration of MDT to all newly detected patients for a number of years.

Several explanations can be advanced for the apparent lack of acceleration of a decline of incidence following the introduction of MDT:
- The long incubation period of leprosy;
- The increased case detection efforts; or
- Detection too late to effect very much of a reduction of transmission.

Immunoprophylaxis

In several randomized controlled trials that have been carried out, vaccination with BCG was shown to reduce the risk of developing leprosy. The level of protection varied among trials from 20–80 percent, for reasons that remain unclear. Repeated vaccination with BCG is capable of enhancing protection against leprosy, and addition of heat-killed *M. leprae* (HKML) to BCG does not appear to increase the protection conferred by BCG alone. However, this has not been true all the trials; in one trial in South India, the combination of BCG + HKML conferred protection that was almost double that conferred by BCG alone. Protection conferred by BCG appears greatly if the vaccine is administered before 15 years of age. The ICRC vaccine was also shown to confer significant protection against leprosy. Current research suggests the possibility of producing vaccines for leprosy that are more effective.

Chemoprophylaxis

Chemoprophylaxis against leprosy has been studied in several trials. A systemic review and meta-analysis of these trials has shown that chemoprophylaxis based on dapsone or intramuscular acedapsone conferred an overall protection against leprosy of about 60 percent. However, the protection appeared to wane over time after administration of the chemo-prophylactic regimen. An uncontrolled trial with rifampicin administered in a single dose at a dosage of 25 mg per kg yielded an estimated protective efficacy of 35–40 percent. Finally, a program of chemoprophylaxis employing single doses of the combination rifampicin-ofloxacin-minocycline, was launched in the Federated States of Micronesia. Kiribati and the Republic of the Marshall Islands as part of their elimination program. Because this was not a controlled trial, but rather an attempt to prevent the disease in an entire population, it is difficult to draw conclusions regarding the degree of protection conferred by this chemoprophylaxis.

Other Factors

Socioeconomic conditions are thought to play an important role in leprosy, their improvement resulting in a decline of incidence. One of the best demonstrations of such an influence was provided by a study of trends of incidence in mainland Japan and Okinawa. Although the factors contributing to this decline are not known, housing conditions, the number of persons per household or per room, and family size are thought to have been most important. A study in Malawi found an inverse relations between the number of years of schooling and the risk of leprosy, and good housing conditions were also associated with a decreased risk of leprosy. Nutritional factors could also influence individual susceptibility.

What are the essential indicators for leprosy epidemiology and control?

Indicators are tools for measuring progress in achieving the objectives of a program. Ideally, these indicators should be valid (measure effectively what they are supposed to measure), simple, easy to measure and to interpret, responsive to changes, and give information that could be used to reorient activities. This section concern the usefulness of a number of indicators often employed in leprosy control programs.

Prevalence

Prevalence should deal with the actual number of people in need of, or receiving therapy. There were several reasons for choosing prevalence, and not incidence, as the indicator of elimination:

- The incidence of leprosy is not easy to measure employing routine reporting systems, which generate information only on case-detection;
- Detection of new cases may correlated very poorly with incidence, because of operational changes in activities;
- Because of the long incubation period, current incidence reflects transmission that had occurred several years earlier and, therefore, does not reflect the effectiveness of current antileprosy activity
- It was hoped that reduction of prevalence to very low levels would lead, in time, to reduction of transmission of infection and, therefore, to reduction of incidence;
- The target of a prevalence of less than 1 in 10, 000 at the national level and the target date of the end of the year 2000, although arbitrary, provided sufficient challenge to build political commitment and intensify activities.

However, prevalence possesses limitations as an indicator of elimination:

- The date collected refers to practice only to those who are registered for treatment. Undetected leprosy patients are not taken into account;
- It is directly dependent upon the duration of treatment;
- Prevalence of registered cases is directly influenced by detection activities, and thus by operational factors.

Incidence

The annual incidence is the number of new cases of a disease that occur in a population in the course of a year. In theory, it represents the best estimate of the current risk of developing leprosy within the specified population. It also reflects the transmission pattern of *M. leprae* in the population during preceding years. However, it is very difficult to measure in practice; clear and undisputed criteria for the diagnosis of leprosy are required, and total populations must be examined at regular intervals. Even in an ideal situation, because some leprosy lesions are evanescent, the number of leprosy patients detected in a program depends upon the frequency at which the population is surveyed.

Even if incidence cannot be measured accurately, its trends can be estimated by set of indicators.

New Case Detection Rate

The rate at which new cases are detected is the most logical proxy-indicator of incidence. However, the new-case detection rate poses some problems of interpretation;

- It is directly influenced by the intensity and frequency of detection activities and the quality of services;
- A number of newly detected cases may have developed leprosy several years earlier;
- At the same time, some people who develop symptoms will be detected only after a number of years, and thus will not be included in the current years' case detection rate.
- In spite of these limitations, one may assume that trends of case detection reflect trends if incidence, on condition that there has been no important change of detection activities, including coverage, self-reporting behavior, diagnostic procedures and criteria.

Proportion of Newly Detected Patients with Grade 2 Impairment

This is highly relevant indicator. The proportions of newly detected patients with impairments have been shown to be related to delay before detection. A large proportion of patients with deformity among newly detected patients indicate that these include old cases, whereas a small and stable proportion of new patients with impairments among the newly detected cases is a sign that the delay between onset of the disease and its diagnosis is stable, and that trends of case detection reflect trends of incidence. However, the validity of this indicator depends upon the thoroughness of the examination of the new patients at the time of detection.

Proportion of Children

A large proportion of children among the newly detected patients is a sign of active and recent transmission of the infection. Thus, it is an important

epidemiological indicators, even though the proportion can also be influenced by operational factors, such as active campaigns among specific sub-groups of the population-school surveys, for example. As transmission of *M. leprae* decreases in a population, the proportion of children among the newly detected cases may also be expected to decrease. However, this is a slow process. Therefore, it would be informative to monitor age-specific case-detection rates or mean age at detection; this should increase in the situation of declining incidence.

Proportion of MB Patients

This indicator is particularly difficult to interpret: the proportion of MB patients among newly detected patients differs from country to country, and is directly influenced by the criteria used for classification (bacteriological or clinical) and by detection efforts. Its usefulness for interpretation of trends of case-detection rates is also questionable: the proportion of MB patients among the newly detected cases has been shown both to increase and to decrease in situation of declining incidence. However, as long as treatment differs for PB and MB patients, the proportion of MB patients will remain useful for estimating drug requirements. It may also be important to collect information on new smear-positive patients; this may be accomplished by the use of 'sentinel' sites.

Treatment Completion Rate

This should be calculated, by cohort analysis, as the proportion of patients who have completed treatment among those expected to do so. As long as treatment differs for PB and MB patients, this indicator must be calculated separately for each type of patient.

Relapses

Although relapses appear to be very rare after MDT, it remains useful to monitor relapse at the program or country level. If a sizeable proportion of the patients starting treatment consist of relapse, the situation is worth investigating.

■ RECOMMENDED READINGS

1. Anonymous. ILEP. The interpretation of epidemiological indicators in leprosy. 25 pp, 2001.
2. Anonymous. WHO. Epidemiology of leprosy in relation to control. Technical Report Series No. 716, Geneva, 1985.
3. Anonymous. World Health Organisation. The final push strategy to eliminate as a public health problem. Questions and answers. First edition, 2002.
4. Anonymous. World Health Organisation Expert Committee on leprosy, Seventh Report, Geneva, 1997.
5. Fine PE, Sterne JA, Ponnighaus JM, Bliss L, Saui J, Chihana A, *et al*. Houshold and dwelling contact as risk factors for leprosy in northern Malawi. *Am J Epidemiol*. 1997;146:91-102.
6. Gupta CM, Tutakne MA, Tiwari VD, Chakrabarty N. Inoculation leprosy subsequent to dog bite. A case report. *Indian J Lepr*. 1984;56:919-920.
7. Noordeen SK. Toward the elimination of leprosy: the challenges and opportunities. *Int J Lepr Other Mycobact Dis*. 1998;66:218-221.
8. Sehgal VN, Inoculation leprosy. Current status. *Int J Dermatol*. 1988;27:6-9.
9. Van Beers SM, Hatta M, Klatser PR. Patient contact is the major determination in incident leprosy: implications for future control. *Int J Lepr Other Mycobact Dis*. 1999;67:119-128.

National Leprosy Eradication Program— Indian Scenario

National Leprosy Eradication Program (NLEP) was launched in the year 1983 with the assistance of World Bank, World Health Organization and many other distinguished international voluntary organizations. It was meant to help eliminate leprosy by the end of year 2000 AD.

The leprosy prevalence rate was estimated at 57 per 10, 000 population in the year 1981. This figure was brought down to 5.2 per 10,000 by March 2000 following the introduction of intensive Multidrug therapy (MDT). 70 percent of leprosy patients in India are in Bihar, Uttar Pradesh, West Bengal, Orissa and Madhya Pradesh. In the course of 1996–1999, two rounds of a modified leprosy elimination campaign (MLEC) were implemented, which resulted in better detection of the disease. It also aimed at promoting public awareness on leprosy, training general health services staff and sensitizing community volunteers to draft them in case detection.

The present appraisal of NLEP, including validation of MLEC-II, was undertaken jointly by WHO, World Bank, the DANIDA leprosy project (DANLEP) and the Government of India between March 27 to April 17, 2000. This exercise was meant to evaluate the progress of NLEP in terms of coverage and achievements, assess the yield of MLEC, as well as the quality of care and accessibility of services. This momentous opportunity was also used to collect information required for the design of the 2nd World Bank project.

On the basis of prevalence rate of leprosy, states were divided into three categories, namely
- Endemic states such as Uttar Pradesh, Madhya Pradesh, Bihar, Orissa and West Bengal,
- Major endemic states Andhra Pradesh, Assam, Gujrat, Karnataka, Kerala, Maharashtra and Tamil Nadu; and
- (So-called) Nonendemic states/union territories: Chandigarh, Delhi, Haryana, Meghalaya, Pondicherry, Punjab, Rajasthan and Tripura.

Primary data was collected from—state leprosy officers (21), district leprosy officers (53), medical officers (239), health assistants (46), non-medical health supervisors (68), multipurpose health workers (95), PMWs (123). Urban households in endemic states (1062), Rural household in endemic states (545), non-endemic states (245). The number of leprosy cases taken for validation of MLEC was 2, 243 from endemic states, 200 from other endemic states and 62 from other nonendemic states.

The several observations brought out during the program are being focused attention to:

EPIDEMIOLOGICAL PROFILE AND LEPROSY TRENDS IN REGISTERED CASES IN INDIA

Trends in registered cases in India: The number of registered leprosy cases per 10, 000 population at the end of the year decreased from 10.7 in March 1994 to 5.2 by March 2000. The percentage of leprosy cases put on MDT also increased from 98.5 percent to 99.7 percent during the same period. It was because of information, education and communication (IEC), accordingly, detection of new leprosy cases per 10, 000 population increased from 5.6 in 1993–94 to 7.0 in 1999–2000.

Trends in leprosy endemicity distribution of districts: The percentage of districts with a registered prevalence rate of > 10 per 10, 000 was 52.8 percent in 1995 in the endemic states of Bihar, West Bengal, Orissa, Uttar Pradesh, Madhya Pradesh. This figure came down to 24.2 percent in 1997 and declined further to 10.8 percent in 1999. Similarly, in the other endemic states such as Andhra Pradesh, Assam, Gujarat, Karnataka, Kerala, Maharashtra and Tamil Nadu the per centage of districts with registered prevalence rate of leprosy > 10 per 10,000 population showed a decline from 8 percent in 1995 to 0.6 percent in the year 1999. The same declining trend was also noted in the nonendemic states of Haryana, Meghalaya, Pondicherry, Punjab, Rajasthan and Tripura, where the percentage of districts with registered prevalence rate of > 10 per 10, 000 population decreased from 3.8 per cent in 1995 to 1.2 percent in 1999.

Trends in new case detection rates: Due to increased IEC activities and other special efforts, the new case detection per year increased from 2,40,383 in 1993 to 4,51,672 in 1999–2000 in the endemic problem states. An increase was recorded also in non-endemic states, from 2,294 in 1993 to 5,489 in 1999–2000.

Trends in percentage of children among new leprosy cases detected: The percentage of children among new leprosy cases detected per year has been in the range of 2.3 percent to 32.9 percent in various states from the year 1993–1994 to 1999–2000.

▌MODIFIED LEPROSY ELIMINATION CAMPAIGN (MLEC) VALIDATION

Suspects, and cases in the sample population detected during MLEC in endemic problem states: In endemic problem states, a sample of 23,832 rural residents and 5,013 urban residents covered under MLEC was screened. The case prevalence rate was 32.3 pcr 10,000 population in rural areas and 35.9 for urban areas. The case prevalence was 47 per 10,000 in males and 37.1 in females, while it was 16.9 in children. It was observed to be higher in under-privileged population groups such as scheduled caste (67.8), scheduled tribes (28.8), and below—the poverty-line groups' (51.9) as compared to other groups' (22.8) per 10,000 population.

Leprosy awareness in communities from the endemic states: 12,193 residents from these states were interviewed to ascertain their awareness level about leprosy. 52–72 percent of the respondents in the endemic states had seen/read/listened to leprosy messages on mass media, 65–75 percent agreed that deformities in leprosy could be prevented through early detection and treatment. 71–84 percent of these respondents enlightened that leprosy patients need not be kept away from the house. The awareness level was observed to be higher in urban areas and among respondents from other castes.

The appraisal teams interviewed 469 community leaders from these states. 59–94 percent of these leaders said they had seen a leprosy case, and 67–89 percent talked about how to detect leprosy in a person. Between 3.6 percent and 66.7 percent of them in various states could fully recount symptoms and signs of leprosy. 15–21 percent of them could not say where MDT/treatment were available. 79–98 percent of these community leaders said they had seen leprosy messages and 48–76 percent had heard of MDT in leprosy. 78–94 percent of the leaders agreed that leprosy could be cured with MDT; 52–91 percent agreed that leprosy-related deformities could be prevented through early detection and treatment.

Leprosy awareness in communities from the other endemic states: 514 residents from these states were interviewed to ascertain their leprosy awareness level. 36–81 percent of them said they had seen a leprosy case, 48–87 percent said they could make out a leprosy suspect. Up to 32.5 percent of the respondents in various states could fully recount leprosy symptoms and signs. 8–33 percent could not say where MDT was available, 60–89 percent of the respondents said they had seen leprosy messages and 20–53 percent had heard of MDT in leprosy. 66–93 percent of the respondents agreed that leprosy could be cured with MDT and 51–91 percent with the statement that leprosy-related deformity could be prevented with early detection and treatment.

Leprosy awareness in communities from non-endemic states: 276 residents from these states were interviewed to ascertain their awareness about leprosy. 4–80 percent of them said they had seen a leprosy case, 39–90 percent said they could suspect leprosy in a victim. 0–41 percent of the respondents in various states could fully recount symptoms and signs of leprosy. 9–83 percent of them could not specify where MDT treatment was available. 36–96 percent of the respondents said they had seen leprosy massages and 8–67 percent had heard of MDT in leprosy. 12–96 percent of the respondents agreed that leprosy could be cured with MDT and 33–80 percent with the statement that leprosy- related deformity could be prevented with early detection and treatment.

MLEC as a case—finding tool for leprosy: In the five endemic problem states, during MLEC-I, a total of 3,76,105 new leprosy cases were reported, and during MLEC-II, 1, 77, 165 new leprosy cases. The other endemic states reported 71, 647 cases during MLEC-I and 39, 596 cases during MLEC-II. From non-endemic states 2,386 new leprosy cases were reported during MLEC-I and 966 during the MLEC-II.

Of the leprosy suspects detected during MLEC campaigns, 67.7 percent were confirmed as leprosy cases by program personnel in endemic problem states, 59 percent in other endemic states and 93 percent in nonendemic states. 84.6 percent of the leprosy cases in endemic problem, 76 percent of the leprosy cases in other endemic states and 78.7 percent of the leprosy cases in nonendemic states were confirmed within seven days of detection.

Appraisal teams confirmed 85–92 percent of the cases diagnosed as leprosy and 86–94 percent of the numbers classified as new leprosy cases by the program during MLEC, in endemic problem states. For the other endemic states the appraisal teams agreed 66–100 percent with the leprosy diagnosis

and 90–100 percent with the leprosy classified. Similar figures for nonendemic states were 66–100 percent and 50–100 percent. The percentage of the recycled cases ranged from 3.6 percent in Madhya Pradesh to 82.4 percent in West Bengal in endemic problem states. The range was from 6.2 percent in Karnataka to 100 percent in Assam among the other endemic states, whereas for nonendemic states the recycled cases reportedly ranged from 33 percent in Haryana to 100 percent in Tripura and Meghalaya.

INFRASTRUCTURE FOR NLEP

The infrastructure for leprosy elimination activities is based on District Leprosy Units, Leprosy Control Units/Modified Leprosy Control Units, Temporary Hospitalization Wards, Sample Survey and Assessment Units, Survey Education and Treatment Units, Mobile Leprosy Treatment Units, Leprosy Rehabilitation Promotion Units, Reconstructive Surgery Units and Leprosy Training Centers. The drug position was observed to be satisfactory in all the states. Good quality MDT drugs were available in sufficient quantities in all parts of the country. The availability of funds and staff was regarded as satisfactory in most states. However, the facilities for disability care, reconstructive surgery, and training for POD need to be strengthened.

RECOMMENDATIONS FOR NLEP IN THE COUNTRY

National leprosy eradication program (NLEP) at the national level has shown considerable progress, in terms of reduction in prevalence rate. However, the progress has been uneven. Some states require special inputs to move faster toward the goal of elimination. The political commitments and bureaucratic support which has been crucial for the program should be continued and further strengthened, especially in high endemic problem states. MDT services are available in the entire districts. It is also encouraging to observe those quality MDT services, accurate diagnosis and classification, fixed duration MDT/treatment, and regular treatment are now being provide in most states. All states have completed training of health personnel for integration of leprosy services with general health services. The five identified endemic states should continue to receive special attention. Integration of leprosy services with general health care should be started; periodic MLEC type activity should be implemented, aiming particularly at the weak and the marginalized; training of general health care staff should be sustained, and IEC should be intensified.

RECOMMENDED READING

1. Bhattacharya SN, Sehgal VN. Leprosy in India. *Clin Dermatol*. 1999;17:159-170.

26

Leprosy—
The Global Scenario

World Health Organization (WHO) and its member-states in the year 1991 committed themselves to eliminate leprosy as a public health problem by the year 2000 AD, elimination being defined as the prevalence of less than one case per 10,000 population.

The latest available information about leprosy across the globe is provided in Table 26.1. It indicates that just a year before the elimination target date, the prevalence rate at the global level is around 1.25 per 10,000 population. Of 122 countries considered endemic in 1985, 98 countries have eliminated the disease. Global prevalence has been reduced by 86 percent. Multidrug therapy (MDT) had cured more than 10 million patients by the end of 1999. The latest available information concerning prevalence and detection country-wise is shown in the Table 26.2.

■ COUNTRIES ENDEMIC FOR LEPROSY

Leprosy remains a public health problem in 24 countries situated mainly in the tropical belt (Population >1 million-prevalence rate >1 case per 10,000 population; and prevalence >100 cases). The top 11 endemic countries have 6,72,596 registered cases and 6,77,086 newly detected cases (Table 26.3). These represent 89 percent of the prevalence and 92 percent of the cases worldwide. India accounts for 67 percent of the prevalence and 73 percent of the detection worldwide. The prevalence rate in these top 11 endemic countries remains 4.1 per 10,000 population, some of these countries may fail in the goal of elimination by 2000 AD despite the intensified efforts being made by national programs.

Table 26.1: Latest available information of prevalence and detection of leprosy, according to WHO region,

WHO region	Cases on treatment (rate per 10, 000)	Number of new cases reported (rate per 100, 000)	Cured with MDT *
Africa	64,490 (1.0)	55,635 (8.6)	6,45,576
Americas	90,447 (1.1)	45,599 (5.7)	256,670
Eastern Mediterranean	8,785 (0.2)	5,757 (1.2)	72,463
Europe	846 (–)	172 (–)	3,683
South-East Asia	574,924 (3.8)	621,620 (41.3)	9507,660
Western Pacific	13,771 (0.1)	9,501 (0.6)	273,161
Total	**753,263 (1.25)**	**738,284 (12.3)**	**10,759,213**

*Cumulative

Table 26.2: Latest available information of registered prevalence of leprosy and detection rate, by WHO region, [a] country-wise.

Country	Registered Cases on 1, January 2000	Prevalence per 10,000	Cases detected during 1999	Detection Rate per 100,000
Africa				
Angola	3,075	2.5	1,840	14.9
Benin	480	0.8	619	10.2
Burkina Faso	940	0.8	879	7.5
Cameroon	1,588	1.1	1,337	9.1
Central African Republic	549	1.5	422	11.8
Chad	749	1.1	1,030	14.5
Congo	464	1.6	53	1.8
Cote d' Ivoire [b]	1,978	1.3	1,719	10.9
Democratic Republic of the Congo [b]	5,031	1.0	4,221	8.6
Ethiopia [b]	7,764	1.3	4,457	7.4
Gambia [b]	132	1.1	115	9.4
Ghana	1,419	0.7	1,620	8.4
Guinea	1,559	2.0	2,475	32.0
Guinea-Bissau	144	1.2	53	4.6
Kenya [b]	546	0.2	233	0.8
Liberia [b]	330	1.0	200	6.0
Madagascar	7,865	4.7	8,704	51.6
Malawi [b]	631	0.5	525	4.5
Mali	1,793	1.5	1,786	14.7
Mozambique	7,403	3.9	5,488	28.7
Niger	2,375	2.3	1,907	18.2
Nigeria	7,707	0.6	7,918	6.3
Senegal	468	0.5	474	5.1
Sierra Leone [b]	1,481	3.1	413	8.5
Uganda	1,180	0.5	888	4.1
United Republic of Tanzania	4,701	1.4	5,081	15.4
Togo	340	0.7	321	7.1
Zambia [b]	768	0.8	198	1.9
Americas				
Argentina	2,000	0.5	471	1.3
Bolivia [b]	116	0.1	73	0.9
Brazil [b]	78,068	4.3	42,055	25.9
Colombia [b]	2,933	0.8	607	1.7

Contd...

Contd...

Costa Rica [b]	142	0.4	13	0.4
Cuba	596	0.5	333	3.0
Dominican Republic [b]	332	0.4	220	2.7
Ecuador [b]	233	0.2	73	0.6
Mexico [b]	2,318	0.2	146	0.1
Paraguay [b]	652	1.2	357	6.7
Peru [b]	262	0.1	63	0.3
Suriname [b]	102	2.3	64	14.6
United States of America [b]	200	0.0	112	0.0
Venezuela	1,334	0.6	771	3.3
Eastern Mediterranean				
Afghanistan	128	0.1	22	0.1
Egypt	3,020	0.5	1,472	2.2
Iran, Islam Republic of [b]	200	0.0	74	0.1
Pakistan	1,905	0.1	927	0.6
Somalia	286	0.3	37	0.4
Sudan	2,332	0.8	2,426	8.3
Yemen	607	0.3	561	3.2
South East Asia				
Bangladesh	11,092	0.9	14,336	11.4
India	4,95,073	5.0	5,37,956	54.3
Indonesia	23,156	1.1	17,477	8.3
Myanmar	28,404	5.9	30,479	62.9
Nepal	13,572	5.7	18,693	78.7
Sri Lanka	1,260	0.7	1,757	9.4
Thailand [c]	2,291	0.4	864	1.4
Western Pacific				
Cambodia	584	0.5	790	7.2
China [b]	4,082	0.0	2,051	0.2
Lao PDR	282	0.5	177	3.2
Malaysia	1,022	0.5	222	1.0
Papua New Guinea	504	1.1	713	15.5
Philippines	4,251	0.6	3,390	4.5
Republic of Korea	551	0.1	21	0.0
Vietnam	2,087	0.3	1,795	2.3

[a] Countries with > 100 cases, [b] Latest available information, [c] Incomplete data.

Table 26.3: Registered prevalence of leprosy and detection rate in the top 11 endemic countries [a]

Country	Registered cases on 1, January 2000	Prevalence per 10,000	Cases detected during 1999	Detection rate per 100,000
India	4,95,073	5.0	5,37,956	54.3
Brazil [b]	78,060	4.3	42,055	25.9
Myanmar	28,404	5.9	30,479	62.9
Indonesia	23,156	1.1	17,477	8.3
Nepal	13,572	5.7	18,693	78.7
Madagascar	7,865	4.7	8,704	51.6
Ethiopia [b]	7,764	1.3	4,457	7.4
Mozambique	7,403	3.9	5,488	28.7
Democratic Republic of the Congo [b]	5,031	1.0	4,221	8.6
United Republic of Tanzania	4,701	1.4	5,081	15.4
Guinea	1,559	2.0	2,475	32.0
Total	**6,72,596**	**4.1**	**6,77,086**	**41.7**

[a] – The top 11 endemic countries *vide supra* have the following characteristics namely; (I) they have a prevalence >1 per 10,000 population; and (ii) the number of prevalent leprosy cases is > 5,000, or the number of newly- detected cases is >2,000. ([b] – 1999 information)

▌LEPROSY TRENDS IN INDIA FROM 1985

Today, India represents 67 percent of the prevalence and 73 percent of the detection worldwide. It is therefore imperative to focus attention on the issue from 1985 onwards (Table 26.4). Prevalence seems to have deceased by 83 percent during the past

Table 26.4: Leprosy trends, India, 1985–1999

End of the year	Prevalence	Prevalence per 10,000	Detection	Detection rate per 100,000
1985	2,916,000	38.6	477,000	63.1
1986	3,017,000	39.1	507,000	65.7
1987	2,962,000	37.6	419,000	65.7
1988	2,835,000	35.3	474,000	56.8
1989	2,633,000	32.1	466,000	56.8
1990	2,130,000	25.5	481,000	57.5
1991	1,673,000	19.6	517,000	60.6
1992	1,167,000	13.4	547,000	62.8
1993	942,000	10.6	494,000	55.6
1994	740,000	8.2	427,000	47.1
1995	573,000	6.2	425,571	46.0
1996	553,793	5.9	415,302	44.0
1997	527,344	5.3	534,411	53.1
1998	577,200	5.9	634,901	64.3
1999	495,073	5.0	537,956	54.3

15 years. It has remained stable ever since 1995. Current prevalence is still at 5 per 10,000 population at the national level. Prevalence, however, at state level ranges from 15 per 10,000 population in Indian state of Bihar, to < 1 per 10,000 in 10 other states. The leprosy disease burden is concentrated mainly in five states namely Bihar, Madhya Pradesh, Orissa, Uttar Pradesh and West Bengal. They account for 70 percent of registered cases together with 70 percent of new cases detected in India. These five states represent 46 percent of registered cases and 51 percent of newly detected cases worldwide. This single fact portrays the magnitude of leprosy in these states, and highlights the importance of effective implementation of intensified elimination strategies.

Leprosy Elimination Campaigns

Leprosy Elimination Campaigns (LECs) is a major development in leprosy programs for the past four years. This 'campaign approach' has improved case detection to a considerable extent. The primary aim of LECs is to bring out hidden cases, patients with established disease but not yet diagnosed and treated. In several public health programs, a campaign approach has been found to be very useful, the polio campaign being a prime example. However, two major questions raised about this approach are its cost-effectiveness and its impact on routine activities. LECs have now been carried out in several countries, some on a small scale, but many on a large scale. The results in terms of detection of new cases appear to be quite impressive. This is also true for India.

What did Leprosy Elimination Campaigns in India Achieved?

— Extracts from a report by Dr CK Rao

Leprosy Elimination Campaigns were introduced by World Health Organization in 1995 as an innovative approach in high endemic areas suspected to harbor many hidden cases. Traditional LECs (on a small scale) were planned for areas with less than half a million population; they were carried out through village visits. Suspected cases of leprosy were detected, and the suspected cases confirmed by leprosy workers before putting them on MDT. Community education was undertaken before and during the campaign activities to promote community awareness and participation.

The traditional pattern of LEC was modified and implemented in India to cover larger areas such as state or country as a whole. Two such MLECs, namely MLEC-I and MLEC-II, were undertaken in India between 1998 and 2000.

MLEC—I Summary of results:

1. About 5,00,000 new leprosy cases detected in the country among three million suspected cases screened.

2. 1/3 of the new cases were of the MB type; 13 percent were single lesion cases (range 4–40 percent) and many of these would not have come for count without an MLEC.

3. Disability rates (Grade – 2) in new cases were below 5 percent.

4. About 20 percent of the suspected leprosy cases did not report for confirmation of diagnosis.

5. Most of the confirmed cases received the first dose of MDT.

6. Some 6,00,000 health staff and 3,50,000 community volunteers were oriented to MLEC related tasks.

7. Concurrent evaluation by the program and subsequent evaluation in selected states by WHO staff/consultant revealed that:

   a. MLEC was a relevant and sound strategy to deal with hidden cases.

   b. Accuracy of diagnosis was over 90 percent; there was an evidence of over diagnosis of single lesion cases.

c. Recycling or re-registration of old cases (partially or fully treated) formed 10–25 percent of the new cases.

d. Under diagnosis was due to non-examination of 10–20 percent of the suspected cases, and early MB a case being missed.

e. MDT drugs of good quality were available at all levels.

f. MDT cure rates were 85–95 percent.

g. New case detection rates did not decline very much 1-year after MLEC.

h. Wide precampaign publicity greatly facilitated community awareness and participation.

MLEC—2 Summary of results:

1. About 1,80,000 new leprosy cases detected in the five states of Bihar, Madhya Pradesh, Orissa, Uttar Pradesh and West Bengal from the screening of 8,00,000 suspected cases.

2. The MB group constituted 38 percent and single lesion cases 10 percent of the new cases.

3. Disability rates in new cases continued to be below 5 percent.

4. Nearly all detected cases received a first dose of MDT.

5. Evaluation of MLEC undertaken as part of an independent program evaluation has brought out the following important findings.

a. Repeat MLEC was justified in the five states.

b. Accuracy of diagnosis was over 90 percent.

c. Recycling/re-registration of old cases namely partially or fully treated among new cases. They accounted for 4 percent of the cases in Madhya Pradesh, 5 percent in Bihar, 26 percent in Orissa, 38 percent in Uttar Pradesh and 82 percent in West Bengal. However, no Plausible explanation available for these variation's.

d. A good quality MDT drug was available at all treatment centers.

LESSONS LEARNT

1. MLECs have enabled improved MDT coverage and better quality of services through active involvement of health centers.

2. Leprosy awareness in the community has increased, leading to better self-reporting of cases even after MLEC.

3. Involvement of health centers during and after MLEC has reduced the social stigma attached to the disease and has improved accessibility and availability of services.

4. Even when implemented well, MLECs may not detect all hidden cases due to one or more of the following reasons:

a. All members of the households are not available during visits.

b. All members present are not willing to be seen by the searchers.

c. Non-reporting of a proportion of suspected cases at confirmation centers.

LECS IN FUTURE

Nation wide MLECs trying to adopt a uniform methodology for the whole country would be inappropriate because of uneven progress in elimination efforts, and varying levels of prevalence. However, in the future, more and more district-specific MLECs should be launched focussing on intensive community education on leprosy and also involving health centers. It is expected that 100 to 150 districts in the country may have to be subjected to MLECs once or twice before the year 2004.

MLECs in future should try to make a distinction between early cases with minimal or doubtful evidence and established cases remaining undetected for long. Secondly, since the magnitude of the problem of recycled old cases showing up, as new detections is uncertain, MLECs should try to identify and exclude them through systematic efforts at eliciting their medical histories. Future MLECs' should also aim at better co-ordination among all agencies concerned with leprosy elimination, including NGOs.

A factual and statistical round-up of leprosy in India and the progress toward leprosy eradication, state by state!

Appendices

Appendix I: Bacteriological Status of Newly Detected Cases

| Classification | Nasal Smear | | | | Cutaneous lesions | | | | |
	+	++	+++	Total	–	+	++	+++	Total
Indeterminate									
Tuberculoid									
Borderline Tuberculoid									
Borderline Borderline									
Borderline Lepromatous									
Lepromatous									
Polyneuritic									
Total									

Appendix II: Classification of Newly Detected Leprosy Cases

Classification	Male			Female			Total
	0–14	15+	Total	0–14	15+	Total	
Indeterminate							
Tuberculoid							
Borderline Tuberculoid							
Borderline Borderline							
Borderline Lepromatous							
Lepromatous							
Polyneuritic							
Total							

Appendix III: Contact Tracing

Index Contact	Contact examined	Lepromatous cases detected among contacts				
		Lepromatous	Indeterminate	Tuberculoid	Unclassified	Total
Indeterminate						
Tuberculoid						
Borderline Tuberculoid						
Borderline Borderline						
Borderline Lepromatous						
Lepromatous						
Polyneuritic						
Total						

Appendix IV: Classification of Disabilities

A. Hands

Grade
  1. Anesthesia to pain.
  2. Mobile claw hand. Useful thumb.
  3. Intrinsic paralysis involving fingers and thumb, or any fingers but with contracture.
  4. Partial absorption of the fingers, but with useful length remaining.
  5. Gross absorption. Stumps only left.

B. Feet

Grade
  1. Anesthesia.
  2. Trophic ulceration (present or past).
  3. Paralysis (foot drop or claw toes).
  4. Partial absorption of the foot (up to one-third of surface area of the sole lost).
  5. Gross absorption (more than one-third of the foot lost).

C. Face

Type
  1. A permanent mark of stigma of leprosy not amounting to ugliness (loss of eyebrows, deformity of the ear).
  2. Collapse of nose.
  3. Paralysis of the eyelids, including lagophthalmos or paralysis of the facial nerve.
  4. Loss of vision in one eye or dimness of vision in both eyes (can count fingers)

D. Miscellaneous

Type
  1. Gynecomastia.
  2. Involvement of the larynx.

Appendix V: Form for Recording Disabilities from Leprosy

Grades	Hand	Foot	Eye	Involvement of larynx
	Sign	LR Sign	LR Sign	LR
Grade 1	Insensitivity Ulcers	Insensitivity	Conjunctivitis	Yes No
	Ulcers and Injuries	Trophic ulcer	Lagophthalmos	
Grade 2	Mobile claw hand	Clawed toes	Iritis or keratitis	Collapse of nose
	Slight absorption	foot drop	YES	No
	Wrist drop	Slight absorption	Blurring of vision	
Grade 3	Stiff joints	Contracture	Severe loss of vision	Facial
	Severe absorption	Severe absorption	Blindness	Paralysis
				Yes No
Maximum grade				

Appendix VI: Leprosy Vaccines

Trials are in progress to develop leprosy vaccines. These are based on the knowledge that mycobacterial cell wall is a powerful adjuvant, capable of potentiating the immune response to a variety of antigens. It stimulates an intense delayed-type hypersensitivity in the host. These vaccines seek to augment the impaired cell-mediated immune response in lepromatous leprosy and/or those at risk of developing it. There are two approaches to the use of these vaccines

1. Immunoprophylaxis, which seeks to prime the immune system to prevent the establishment of infection.
2. Immunotherapy which seeks to boost the suboptimal cell-mediated response in order to prevent the development of severe forms of the disease.

The various vaccines undergoing trials are:

1. BCG
2. Heat killed *M. leprae*
3. BCG and heat killed *M. leprae* derives from armadillo.
4. ICRA vaccine developed at the Cancer Research Institute (CRI). The ICRA bacillus belongs to the *M. avium intercellular* group and is inactivated by γ-irradiation.
5. Vaccine developed at National Institute of Immunology (NII), New Delhi from soil mycobacterium (*M. w*).
6. Vaccine developed at Central Drug Research Institute in Lucknow from *Mycobacterium habana* is also a candidate for inclusion in the trial.

Research is in progress to develop synthetic vaccines based on specific antigens or antigens subunits. By using shuttle plasmid, it has been possible to introduce foreign DNA into cultivable mycobacteria. This represents the first step in the development of engineered cultivable mycobacteria, such as BCG, as vaccine vehicles to express protective antigens for *M. leprae*.

Although effective immuno-prophylaxis would be ideal yet, there is very little data to support the efficacy of currently available vaccines.

Appendix VII: Animal Models for Mycobacterium Leprae

Mycobacterium leprae, the presumptive causative organism of leprosy, has thus far not been cultured *in vitro*. All the knowledge about it has resulted from its cultivation in various animals. The animal cultivation helps in:
1. Establishing the genuinness of any claim of supposed culture of *M. leprae in vitro*.
2. Screening of antileprosy drugs.
    a. Detection of active drug.
    b. Characterization of the effects of active drug.
    c. Monitoring of antibacterial effects in human trial.
    d. Detection of persister.
    e. Detection of drug resistant bacilli.
    f. Clarification of therapeutic problems in leprosy.
3. Determination of the viability of the lepra bacilli.

An ideal animal model for cultivating *M. leprae* should be:
*   Available in large numbers
*   Easy to maintain
*   Viable economically
*   Capable of breeding in captivity
*   Body temperature similar to man
*   Long life span as the incubation period of leprosy is long
*   Should be able to reproduce the spectrum of leprosy after inoculation, which should clinically resemble the infection in man.

Though various animal models have been put forward, the important once are:
1. Footpad of mice
2. Thymectomized, irradiated immunosuppressed mice
3. Nine-banded armadillo
4. Neonatally thymectomized rats
5. Congenital athymic nude mice
6. Mangabey monkey
7. Indian pangolin
8. Slender=Loris
9. Korean chipmunks
10. European hedgehog.

The various animal model were developed as none of them satisfied all the criteria of an ideal animal model.

Footpad of mice: It is the first animal model, developed by sheperd in 1960, 85 years after the discovery of *M. leprae* by Hansen. He reported self-limiting localized multiplication of *M. leprae* in footpad of mice. However, it has certain limitations, namely:
1. Unaltered, mouse foes not provide adequate quantities of lepra bacilli.
2. Shorter life span and thus not suitable for study of characteristic of leprosy.

Immuno-supressed mice: Rees (1966) and Rees et al (1967) introduced immuno-suppressed (thymectomized and/ or irradiated) mice. It resulted in generalized infection similar to that produces in highly susceptible people who suffer from lepromatous leprosy. However, its disadvantages are:
1. The spectrum of leprosy seen in man is not reproduced in the immunosuppressed mice. All immunosuppressed mice develop generalized infection while in man, only a few percent develop generalized disease.

2. In immunosuppressed mice there is a generalized suppression of cell-mediated immunity (CMI), while in lepromatous leprosy, the depression of immunity has been regarded as specific for *M. leprae*. The nonspecific CMI recovers after treatment.
3. Quantity of lepra bacilli produced is less.
4. The disposition of dapsone in mouse is much different from that in man and thus chemotherapeutic studies performed in mouse model have only limited application to the treatment of leprosy in man.

Armadillo: It is considered to be favorable model as:

1. It reacts to lepra bacilli in the same way as man. On inoculation of *M. leprae*, unless one overwhelms the animals' immunity by infecting exceedingly high numbers, only some animals develop the disease. Thus on infection, the armadillos respond with spectrum of leprosy.
2. Armadillo has a longer life span of 15 years, and is thus suitable for leprosy which has long incubation period.
3. The yield of *M. leprae* is large.

The limitations of armadillo are:

1. The animal is found only in America.
2. The animal does not breed readily in captivity.
3. Expensive to maintain animal in laboratory.
4. Housing area must be temperature controlled to 25° C.
5. The yield of lepra bacilli is enormous and thus a potential threat for its attendants, as large number of bacilli are released in the environment and may cause infection through respiratory tract.

Appendix VIII: Early Diagnosis: Newer Techniques

The diagnosis of leprosy is primarily clinical and is based on well-defined clinical criteria. Treatment should be initiated only when the diagnosis is unequivocal. Laboratory aids, facilitating the early diagnosis of suspicious lesion are nonproductive and uncalled for. Moreover, none of the tests developed so far are specific/sensitive. Furthermore, they are expensive and their application in leprosy control program is doubtful. Nonetheless, it is imperative to be aware of these newer techniques.

a. The assay for antiphenolic glycolipid-1 (PGL-1) antibodies, directed against highly specific antigen of *M. leprae* is a well-formed test. It has been evaluated for its usefulness in diagnosis of preclinical cases, the cardinal expression of which is a nondescript bizarre, hypopigmented 'macule' with nonspecific histology. Although a positive test may confirm the diagnosis, yet a negative result does not exclude its possibility.

b. Polymerase chain reaction (PCR) is a sensitive test for detection of *M. leprae* specific antigens. However, its cost and technical intricacies limit its usefulness.

c. Immunocytochemical techniques and special staining procedures may facilitate the detection of neural involvement and an acid-fast bacillus (AFB) is tissue section.

Appendix IX: Standard Protocol

Registration   O.P.D. No.

Name   Age/Sex

Permanent Address

Native Place

Stay in last 10 years

Occupation

Present Illness

Ulcers & blisters

Numbness

Epistaxis

Formication

Anesthesia

Pain

Fever

Deformities

Age of onset of disease

Factors responsible for acute phases if any

Past History

Family History   Relationship   Age

     Father

     Mother

     Brother

     Sister

Extra-Familial

Personal History

Accommodation Facilities

No. of Rooms

No. of people living

General Examination

Facies

General Nutrition   Good/Fair/Bad

Anemia

Jaundice

Eyes   Right

     Left

Nose   Right Nostril

     Left Nostril

     Bridge of Nose

Ear

Eyebrows

Edema

Gynaecomastia

Pulse

Temperature

Blood Pressure

Lymphadenopathy

Local Examination

Type of lesion	Macule/Pauls/Plaque/Nodule		
Erythema/hypopigmented/hyperpigmented			
Margins-well defined/ill-defined			
Regular irregular			
Surface-smooth/rough/shiny/dry			
Scaly/non-scaly			
Flat/raised			
Induration-Peripheral/Central/Whole lesion/None			
Sweating-Present/Absent/Impaired			
Number	1–3		
	10		
	20		
	Numerous	Uncountable	
Distribution—Symmetrical/Asymmetrical/Localised/Others			
Hairs			
Sensory functions of the affected area			
	Normal	Impaired	Absent
Temperature			
Touch			
Pain			
Nerves	Right		Left

Greater auricular Nerve
Ulnar Nerve
Median Nerve
Radial Nerve
Lateral Popliteal Nerve
Posterior tibial Nerve
Others
Systemic Examination
Cardiovascular system
Respiratory system
Digestive system
Lymphatic system
Central Nervous system
Provisional Diagnosis
7 Group Classification
Indeterminate (I)
Tuberculoid (TT)
Borderline Tuberculoid (BT)
Borderline Borderline (BB)
Borderline Lepromatous (BL)
Lepromatous (LL)
Polyneuritic (P)
Ridley and Jopling Classification
Tuberculoid (TT)
Borderline Tuberculoid (BT)
Borderline Borderline (BB)
Borderline Lepromatous (BL)
Lepromatous (LL)

Investigations

Bacteriological Examination

Sites	Number of (+)
Skin-I	
Skin-II	
Skin-III	
Skin-IV	
Earlobe-I	
Earlobe-II	
Nasal Mucosa-I	
Total Number of (+)	

Bacteriological Index = Total No. f (+) No. of sites

Blood Examination

Hb	TLC	DLC	ESR

Histopathologic Examination

Immunological Investigations

Lepromin Testing	48 hours (Fernandez)		After 4 wks. (Mitsuda)
	0		0
	+1		+1
	+2		+2
	+3		+3

Hematology	Percentage		Absolute
Total lymphocyte count			
T cell counts			
T_4 (Helper/Inducer)			
T_5 (Suppressor/Cytotoxic)			
B cell count			
Tissue section			
Absolute lymphocyte count			
T cell counts			
T_4 (Helper/Inducer)			
T_5 (Suppressor/Cytotoxic)			
B cell count			

Appendix X: Vocabulary of Generic and Trade Names of the Drugs and Their Availability

Generic	*Trade Names*
Acetylsalicylic acid	Aspirin, 300 mg (tablet)
	Acetylsalicylic acid, 300 mg (tablet)
Amithiozone	Thiacetazone, 50 mg (tablet)
Analgin	Analgin, 500 mg (tablet)
Atropine sulfate	Atropin sulfate
	1 percent (ointment)
	1 percent (drops)
Betamethasone	Celestone, 0.5 mg (tablet)
	Betnesol, 0.5 mg (tablet)
	Betnelan, 0.5 mg (tablet)
	Betacortil, 0.5 mg (tablet)
Chloramphenicol	Chloromycetin, 100 mg (capsule)
	Reclor, 500 mg (capsule)
Chloroquin diphosphate	Chloroquin, 150 mg (tablet)
	Resochin, 250 mg (tablet)
Clofazimine	Lamprene, Hansepran,
	50 mg 10 mg (capsule)
Cycloserine	Cycloserine, 250 mg (capsule)
	Cyclorin, 250 mg (capsule)
Cyclandelate	Cyclospasmol, 200 mg (tablet)
Dexamethasone	Decadron, 0.5 mg (tablet)
	Dexona, 0.5 mg (tablet)
Diaminodiphenyl sulfone	Dapsone, 50 mg (pink tablet) *
	Dapsone, 100 mg (white tablet) *
	Novophone, 10 mg (tablet)
	Novophone, 25 mg (tablet)
	Novophone, 50 mg (tablet)
	Novaphone, 100 mg (tablet)
	Siosulphone, 25 mg (tablet)
	Siosulphone, 50 mg (tablet)
	Siosulphone, 100 mg (tablet)
Diacetyldiaminodiphenyl sulfone	Acedapsone, 225 mg (ampule)
Disodium hydrogen citrate	Citralka, 114 ml (bottle)
	Citralka, 450 ml (bottle)
	Alkacit, 114 ml (bottle)
	Alkacit, 450 ml (bottle)
Ethionamide	Ethionamide, 125 mg (tablet)
Framycetin sulfate	Soframycin, 1 percent (Cream)
Framycetin sulfate (1 percent) 7	Sofracort eye drops
Hydrocortisone acetate (1.16 percent)	

Gentamicin sulfate	Genticyn, 40 mg/ml (ampule)
	Garamycin 40 mg/ml (ampule)
Glucosulphone sodium	Promin, 5 mg (ampule)
Hydrocortisone acetate	Efcorlin, 1 percent (drops)
	Efcorlin, 1 percent (Ointment)
Isoxsuprine hydrochloride	Duvadilan, 10 mg (tablet)
Isonicotinic acid hydrazide	Isonex, 50 mg (tablet)
	Isonex, 100 mg (tablet)
	Isonex Forte, 300 mg (tablet)
	Isoniazid, 100 mg (tablet)
Minocyclin	Minocycline, 100 mg (tablet)
Neomycin sulfate	Neomycin sulfate, 10 gm
3.5 mg per gram	Neomycin sulfate, 15 gm (tube)
Nylidrin hydrochloride	Arlidin, 6 mg (tablet)
Oxytetracycline	Oxytetracycline
Hydrochloride	hydrochloride, 250 mg (capsule)
	Terramycin, 250 mg (capsule)
Oflaxacin	Tarivid, 200 mg
	Tarivid, 400 mg (tablet)
Para-aminosalicylic acid	PAS 70 percent, 100 g pack
	PAS sodium, 500 mg (tablet)
Paracetamol	Crocin, 500 mg (tablet)
Pefloxacin	Pelox, 400 mg (tablet)
	Metacin, 500 mg (tablet)
Polymyxin B sulfate (5000 u)	
Potassium antimony tartrate	
Zinc bacitracin (400 u)	
Zinc sulfadiazine	Zad-G (cream)
Neomycin sulfate (3400 u)	Neosporin
Prednisolone	Prednisolone, 5 mg (tablet)
	Wysolone, 5 mg (tablet)
	Hostacortin-H, 5 mg (tablet)
Pyrazinamide	Pyrazinamide, 500 mg (tablet)
Rifampicin	Rifacilin, 150 mg (capsule)
	Rifacilin, 300 mg (capsule)
	Rifacilin, 450 mg (capsule)
	Rifacin, 150 mg (capsule)
Solapsone	Sulphetron, 500 mg (tablet)
Stibophen, 64 mg/ml	Fantorin, 25 ml (vial)
Sulfapyridine	Sulfapyridine, 500 mg (tablet)
	MB 693, 500 mg (tablet)
Xantinol nicotinate	Complamina, 150 mg (tablet)
	Complamina retard, 150 mg (tablet)

Index

KOBE BRYANT

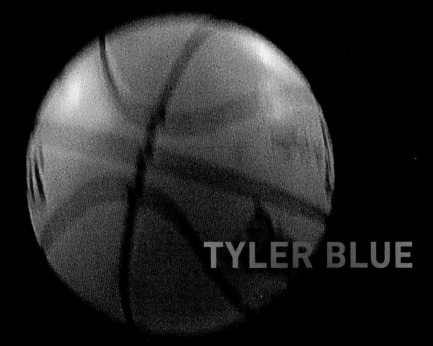

TYLER BLUE

Abbeville Kids
An Imprint of Abbeville Press
New York London

Project editor: Lauren Orthey
Copy editor: Jennifer Dixon
Layout: Ada Rodriguez
Production manager: Louise Kurtz

Illustrations by Pavel Shevelev: pp. 9, 11, 13, 15, 17, 19, 21, 23 (and back cover middle)

PHOTOGRAPHY CREDITS

Alamy: front cover (Action Plus Sports Images); p. 25 (© Ron Tarver/KRT/ABACA); p. 27 (© Bruce Cotler/Globe Photos/ZUMAPRESS.com); p. 29 (Rich Kane Photography); p. 30 (UPI/Lori Shepler); p. 33 (UPI); p. 41 and back cover top (Chris Carlson/KRT/ABACA); p. 42 (Zuma Press, Inc.); p. 47 and back cover bottom (UPI Photo/Jim Ruymen); p. 48 (Gouhier-Hahn-Nebinger/Cameleon/ABACAPRESS.com); p. 49 (UPI Photo/Roger L. Wollenberg); p. 55 (Image Press Agency); p. 56 (ZUMA Press, Inc.); p. 57 (UPI Photo/Jim Ruymen); p. 59 (European Sports Photo Agency); p. 61 (© Burt Harris/Prensa Internacional/ZUMAPRESS.com); pp. 62–63 (UPI/John Angelillo)

Icon Sportswire: p. 6 (Ray Grabowski); p. 31 (Matt A. Brown); p. 35 (John W. McDonough), p. 39 (John W. McDonough/SI); p. 40 (Kevin Reece); pp. 44–45 (Icon Sports Media); p. 50 (Christophe Elise/DPPI); p. 51 (Christophe Elise/DPPI); p. 53 (Icon Sportswire)

Imago Images: p. 2 (Photo News); p. 7 (ZUMA Press Wire); p. 36 (ZUMA Press Wire); p. 37 (ZUMA Press Wire); p. 43 (ZUMA Press Wire)

Please note: This book has not been authorized by the Kobe Bryant estate.

First edition
10 9 8 7 6 5 4 3 2 1

Library of Congress Cataloging-in-Publication Data
Names: Blue, Tyler author
Title: Kobe Bryant / Tyler Blue.
Description: First edition. | New York : Abbeville Kids, An Imprint of
   Abbeville Press, [2025] | Series: Abbeville sports | Audience term:
   juvenile | Audience: Ages 9–12 Abbeville Press. | Audience: Grades 4–6
   Abbeville Press. | Summary: "An illustrated book about Kobe Bryant's
   life and career" —Provided by publisher.
Identifiers: LCCN 2025003386 | ISBN 9780789215109 hardcover
Subjects: LCSH: Bryant, Kobe, 1978–2020—Juvenile literature. | Basketball
   players—United States—Biography—Juvenile literature.
Classification: LCC GV884.B794 B58 2025 | DDC 796.323092
   [B]--dc23/eng/20250130
LC record available at https://lccn.loc.gov/2025003386

For bulk and premium sales and for text adoption procedures, write to Customer Service Manager, Abbeville Press, 655 Third Avenue, New York, NY 10017, or call 1-800-Artbook.

Visit Abbeville Kids online at www.abbevillefamily.com.

CONTENTS

On January 13, 1999, an epic chapter in NBA history closed on a frigid Chicago day. Throngs of reporters packed the United Center—home of the Chicago Bulls—to hear Michael Jordan announce, for the second time in his storied career, his retirement from the game of basketball.

In October 1993, a 30-year-old Jordan had shocked the world by abruptly and unexpectedly stepping away from the game, fresh off leading the Bulls to their third straight championship and in the prime of his career. About one and a half years later, Jordan went back to the Bulls and quickly returned to the apex of the NBA hierarchy, leading Chicago to championships in 1996, 1997, and 1998.

This time, though, nobody was surprised. The Jordan Era was finished.

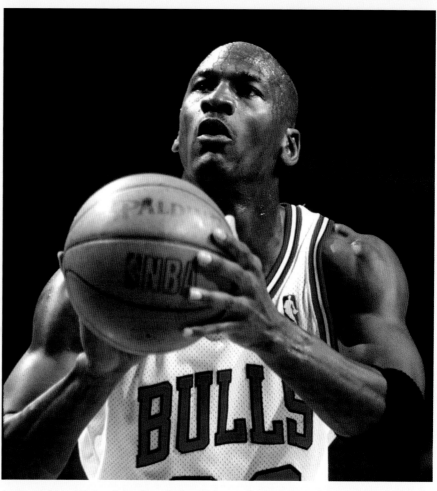

Late 1990s: Michael Jordan of the Chicago Bulls gets ready to shoot.

Jordan dominated the game of basketball like few athletes have ever dominated their sport. In the 1990s, his Bulls won six championships in eight years. Jordan was a five-time League MVP, led the league in scoring 10 times, and was a larger-than-life figure whose star power transcended the sport and made him one of the most popular and marketable celebrities in the world.

With Jordan at the helm, the NBA soared. Just a few months earlier, in June 1998, a record 36 million people had tuned in to Game 6 of the

NBA Finals and watched in awe as, in the final seconds of the game, Jordan stole the ball from future Hall-of-Famer Karl Malone of the Utah Jazz before hitting the game-winning shot at the other end of the court to secure his sixth and final championship.

That was then. Now, the NBA was mired in a months-long lockout that had delayed the start of the 1998–99 season. Some thought the whole season was in jeopardy. The lockout, which came about because the millionaire athletes and the billionaire owners couldn't come

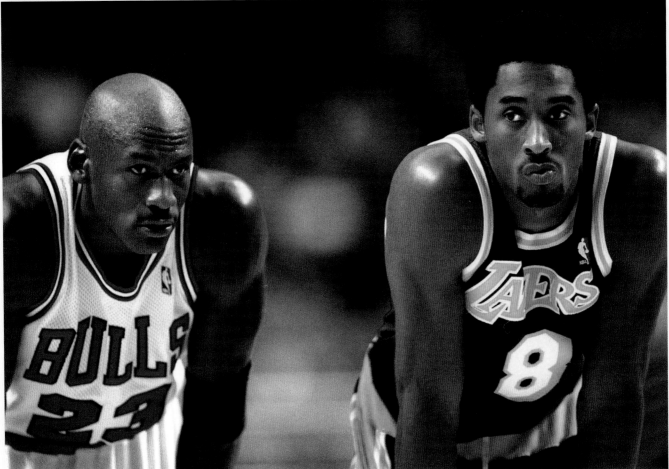

1997: Two basketball legends—Jordan and Kobe Bryant—on the court during free throws

to terms on a collective bargaining agreement, strained the relationship between the league and its fans.

On top of that, the NBA was now losing its superstar. All of a sudden, the league's future looked uncertain. It desperately needed a new star to fill Jordan's sizeable shoes and lead it into the twenty-first century. But who could possibly replicate Jordan's skill and force of personality?

Though many young stars would jockey for the title of Jordan's heir, such as the Philadelphia 76ers Allen Iverson and the Toronto Raptors

Vince Carter, the answer came from a somewhat unlikely source. Over the next few years, a 20-year-old with a memorable name and unlimited confidence in his ability would emerge as the new face of the NBA.

The 1990s indeed belonged to Michael Jordan. But the '90s were over. The next decade, as everybody was about to find out, would belong to Kobe Bean Bryant.

KOBE BEAN

Kobe Bean Bryant entered the world on August 23, 1978, in Lower Merion Township, Pennsylvania, an affluent suburb located just outside of Philadelphia. The son of Joe and Pam Bryant, Kobe had basketball in his blood. Joe hailed from Philadelphia and in the early 1970s was widely regarded as the best player in the Philadelphia Public League while suited up for Bartram High School.

Though he stood 6'9" and played the center position, Joe didn't play the game like a traditional "big man." In those days, centers were expected to camp out close to the basket, post up, and use their height to shoot short shots over their opponents. That didn't suit Joe, who liked to play more like a guard, bringing the ball up the court and mesmerizing the crowd with dizzying displays of ballhandling, flashy passes, and outside shooting. Joe liked to play with flair.

A silky-smooth athlete on the court, Joe earned the nickname "Jellybean," inspired by an old Glenn Miller song: "It Must Be Jelly ('Cause Jam Don't Shake Like That)." Colleges across the country lined up for Jellybean's services. In the end, though, he decided to stay local and committed to La Salle University.

Pam's side of the family was no slouch in the athletics department either. Her brother, John Arthur "Chubby" Cox III, a 6'2" guard, played college ball at Villanova before transferring to the University of San Francisco. He had a brief stint in the NBA. Pam herself stood 5'10" and played her share of basketball growing up. "I hear she has a mean jump shot," Kobe once said of his mother.

As a junior at La Salle, Joe averaged 21.8 points and 11.4 rebounds per game, impressive numbers that convinced him he was ready for the NBA. He decided to skip his senior year, and the Golden State Warriors selected him as the 14th pick of the 1975 NBA draft. However, because of an inexplicable clerical error, the Warriors never sent Joe a contract, and he became a free agent. The Philadelphia 76ers jumped at the chance to sign the local legend. Once again, Jellybean was staying home.

Back then, the Sixers held their preseason training camp at locations west of Philadelphia. The drive from the city to camp took Joe past a restaurant called Kobe Japanese Steak House, which became a popular hangout for Sixers players. Joe in particular grew fond of the place.

When Joe was entering his fourth NBA season in 1978, his wife was pregnant with their third child and first son. The couple sensed their son would be special and wanted to give him a unique name. Joe knew just what it should be. They would name their son Kobe.

Late 1970s: Joe "Jellybean" Bryant, Kobe's dad, dunks a basketball while playing for the Philadelphia 76ers.

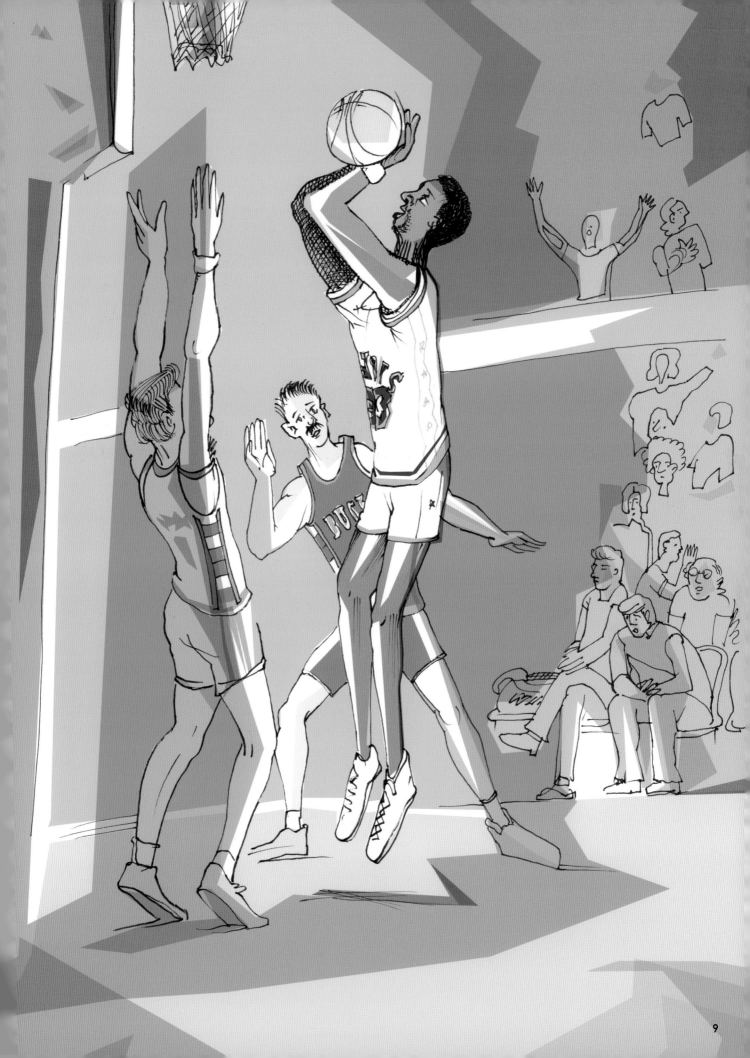

FAMILY MATTERS

Together, Joe and Pam built a tight-knit family. Fittingly, the two had met at a basketball game. Joe, then a sophomore at La Salle, had scored 19 points and pulled down 15 rebounds in the Explorers' blow-out win over Lehigh at the Palestra, a historic basketball arena in Philadelphia, to open the 1973–74 season.

Pam Cox happened to be at that game, which was the first of a doubleheader. Following the La Salle-Lehigh game was a matchup between Villanova and Richmond. Pam's brother, John, played for Villanova, and Pam made the trek from Pittsburgh, where she attended Clarion State, to watch her brother's game.

In between the two games, Joe ran into Pam. The pair struck up a conversation and went on their first date that very night. Within a year they were married. During Joe's rookie season with the 76ers in March 1976, Pam gave birth to a daughter named Sharia. Sixteen months later, Sharia became a big sister with the birth of Shaya. Their baby brother came a year after that.

As their little brother's star grew, Sharia and Shaya took it upon themselves to protect him. With Sharia standing at 5'10" and Shaya at 6'2", they surely made for a formidable presence. Athletes in their own right, both of Kobe's big sisters would go on to play college volleyball, Sharia at Temple and Shaya at La Salle.

Early on in Kobe's life, the Bryants spent so much time at the 76ers' basketball arena, known as the Spectrum, that it was practically their second home. But Joe's career didn't progress as he had hoped, and Philadelphia traded him to the San Diego Clippers in 1979. He was later traded to the Houston Rockets, who declined to renew his contract following the 1982–83 season.

No other team showed any interest in Joe. At the ripe old age of 28, his time in the NBA had come to an end. He was trying to make sense of his new life as a car salesman when an opportunity arose to continue his professional basketball career in Europe. The more Joe and Pam learned about it, the better it sounded. The money was good and the schedule much less demanding than in the U.S., which meant Joe could spend more time with his wife and kids.

In 1984, the Bryants moved to Rieti, Italy, a town of about 40,000 located an hour northeast of Rome. Though five-year-old Kobe and his older sisters picked up Italian quickly—the three would practice together every day after school—the family found it difficult at first to make friends in this new country. So they turned to each other. Already close as a family, those years in Italy helped develop even stronger bonds between them as they traveled around Europe together.

Early 1980s: A young Kobe has a tight-knit family, and especially loves playing with sisters Sharia and Shaya.

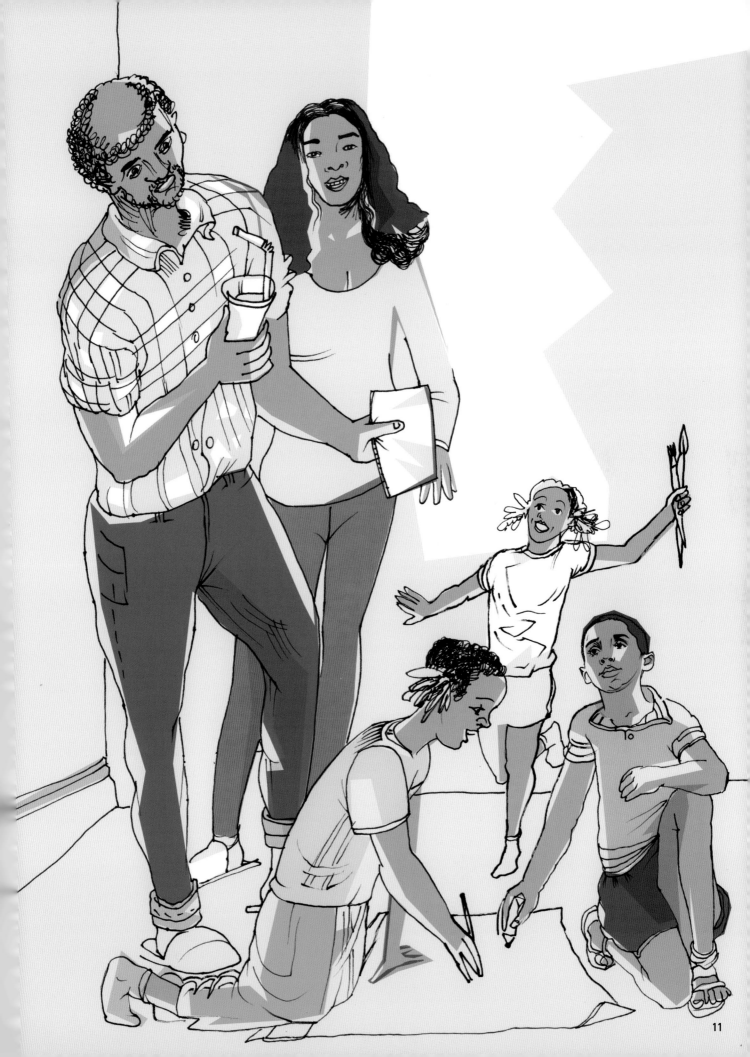

LIKE FATHER,

At one end of the hallway, a small trampoline stands in front of a miniature basketball hoop. At the other stands a three-year-old Kobe Bryant, clutching a kid-sized basketball. The toddler runs down the hallway, a look of pure joy on his face as he hops onto the trampoline, springs into the air, and jams the ball in the hoop. His mother admonishes him, warning he will break the hoop. It has no effect on the young boy, who picks up the ball and slams it again.

Kobe relished everything about having a professional basketball player for a father. He loved going to the games; he loved the way the crowd reacted whenever Jellybean made a play; he loved trying to mimic the moves he saw his father make. While attending school in San Diego during the time Joe played for the Clippers, Kobe would give his teacher updates on his father's exploits of the night before as if he were a sportscaster on the nightly news.

In Italy, NBA games were rarely broadcast on television, and so Kobe's grandparents would periodically record the games and send the tapes to Italy. Kobe would watch—no, *study*—the games diligently. Often, his father would watch with him, analyzing each play and explaining what was going on. Kobe developed a particular fascination with Earvin "Magic" Johnson, the 6'9" point guard of the Los Angeles Lakers, who was redefining what big men in basketball were capable of.

Joe, who had a similar skillset, wasn't quite as impressed. "He comes into the league with all that stuff, and they call it magic," Joe once said of Johnson. "I've been doing it all these years, and they call it 'schoolyard.'" Suffice to say, Joe felt the NBA hadn't fully appreciated him or given him a fair shake. Kobe internalized his father's frustrations and vowed to redeem the Bryant name, no matter what it took.

In terms of national prestige, basketball placed a distant second to soccer in Italy. While Kobe played "the beautiful game" of soccer and enjoyed it, basketball was his passion. But he often found it difficult to convince his friends to take a break from the soccer field to join him on the hardwood. No problem. Kobe invented a game called "shadow basketball," which involved him playing entire games by himself against imaginary opponents.

While shadow ball may have helped young Kobe's visualization skills, it couldn't compare to playing on an actual team. So Joe signed his son up for a club team. Throughout Europe, organized sports are run by clubs. For example, one basketball club will sponsor several teams across different age groups, from youth to adult.

In Kobe's first game, he dribbled and shot so much—scoring the first 10 points of the game—that his teammates were in tears for being ignored. Their parents yelled at the coach to get Kobe off the court. When the coach finally did send Kobe to the bench, Kobe began sobbing, running to Pam's side for comfort. One thing was for certain: the kid could play.

Late 1980s: Kobe plays "shadow basketball"—a game against imaginary opponents—to perfect his skills.

LIKE SON

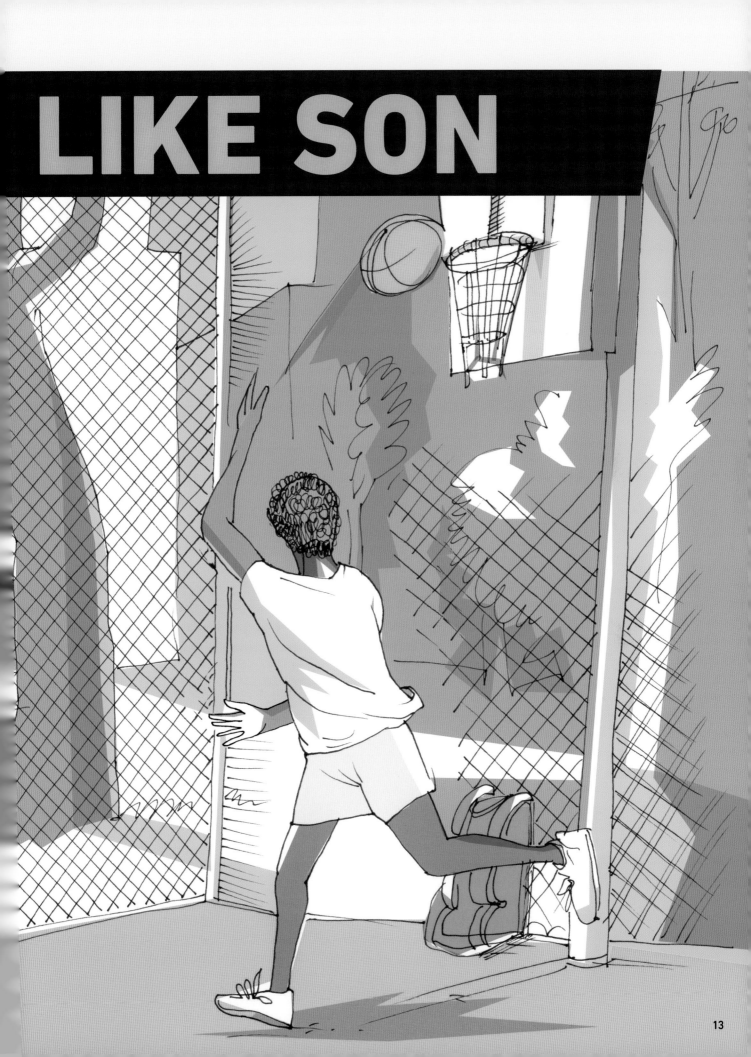

ONE-TRACK MIND

Soon after Kobe started playing organized basketball in Italy, it became quite obvious he had inherited his father's prodigious talent. Before long, Kobe was among the best players of any age in his club. While he might have inherited his father's skills, his personality was all Pam's.

To be sure, it takes a certain personality type for the nickname "Jellybean" to stick. Joe was an affable man, taking time to say hello and chat with everybody he met. He also had a reputation for being a bit of a goofball, someone who could have perhaps benefited from taking his career a little more seriously. Pam, though, was serious enough for both of them. While her husband was out "playing," she ran the household and dished out the discipline. She made sure Kobe got his schoolwork done before he worked on his game, and she made it clear that good grades were a prerequisite for extracurriculars.

On the court, Kobe mirrored his mother's seriousness, hardly ever smiling during games. And why should he? He wasn't there to play nice or make friends. He was there to prove he was the best basketball player around—period. At a young age, Kobe set a goal not only to play professional basketball but also to become the greatest player of all time. Everything he did was in pursuit of those goals.

This single-mindedness often came at the expense of his social life. As he grew up, he cared next to nothing about hanging out with friends, attending parties, and dating. He did care about studying game film, memorizing the moves of professionals such as his father, Michael Jordan, and Magic Johnson, and then spending countless hours on the court incorporating what he observed into his own repertoire.

He had a basketball in his hand so often, Pam would refer to it as his "girlfriend." At one point in high school, Kobe had something close to an actual girlfriend. He started spending time with a girl named Jocelyn Ebron. More often than not, their "dates" consisted of Jocelyn coming over to Kobe's house, sitting next to him on the couch, and watching videos of old basketball games. For some reason, they didn't last.

But Kobe understood the difficulty of accomplishing the goals he had set for himself, and he knew perfectly well how hard he had to work if he was serious about reaching them. And if Kobe was anything, he was serious. He was Pam Bryant's son, after all.

Early 1990s: In Italy, Kobe develops a love for basketball by playing with a youth club team.

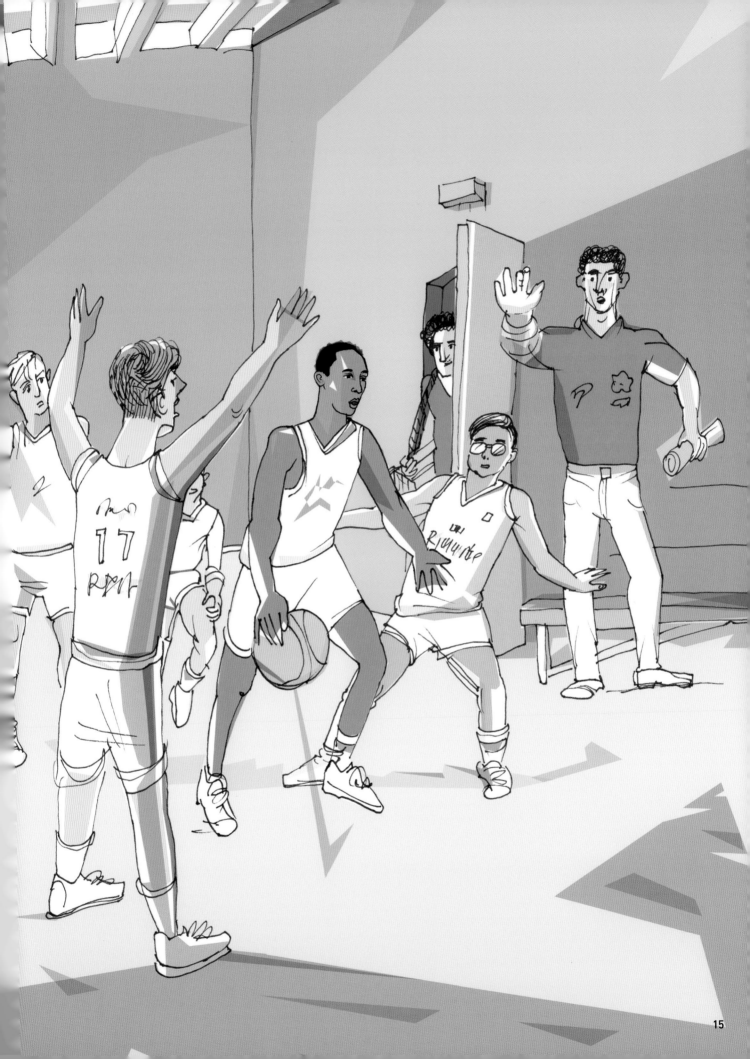

BACK TO AMERICA

Joe Bryant carved out an incredibly successful career in Italy. Against admittedly inferior talent, Jellybean excelled. At the time, very few players in Europe could match his blend of size, skill, and athleticism, and he was finally allowed to play the game the way he wanted, initiating the offense, dishing out flashy assists, and shooting outside shots. Soon, he earned a new nickname: "the Show."

But by 1991, time was catching up with him. He had just finished his 16th season of professional basketball, and he had lost a step or two. Meanwhile, Kobe's game was starting to blossom. Already over six feet tall, Kobe towered above most of his classmates. Although still middle-school-aged, he could already dunk a basketball with ease. When Kobe played one-on-one games against his father, Joe had to actually try in order to win. Kobe's desire to become the best basketball player of his generation still burned strongly. But to be the best, he had to play the best, and the best players were in America.

So Joe decided to retire, and in November 1991, the Bryants relocated to the U.S. It was time for Joe to turn his attention to his son's development. They moved to a town called Wynnewood, an affluent suburb of Philadelphia, and Kobe enrolled as an eighth grader at Bala Cynwyd Middle School.

Adjusting to life in the States was much more difficult for 13-year-old Kobe than adjusting to life in Italy had been eight years prior. He didn't have as good a grasp of the English language as his peers and knew none of the slang. He didn't know the "cool" way to dress or who the popular music artists and celebrities were. But on the basketball court, Kobe could speak a sort of universal language.

Word that the new student was the son of a former NBA player soon got around, and one day a classmate challenged Kobe to a game of one-on-one. When Kobe arrived at the court after school, he was surprised to see dozens of students gathered around to watch. They wouldn't soon forget what they witnessed.

Kobe completely demolished his challenger, proving to be superior in every way. His years of playing club ball in Italy had given him sound fundamentals his opponent lacked; his talent and will to win took care of the rest. The game culminated with Kobe driving by his opponent and—to the shock and glee of all those spectators—dunking the ball through the hoop. Kobe Bryant now had his classmates' attention—and their respect.

Early 1990s: Back in the United States, Kobe impresses his Bala Cynwyd Middle School classmates with his impressive basketball skills.

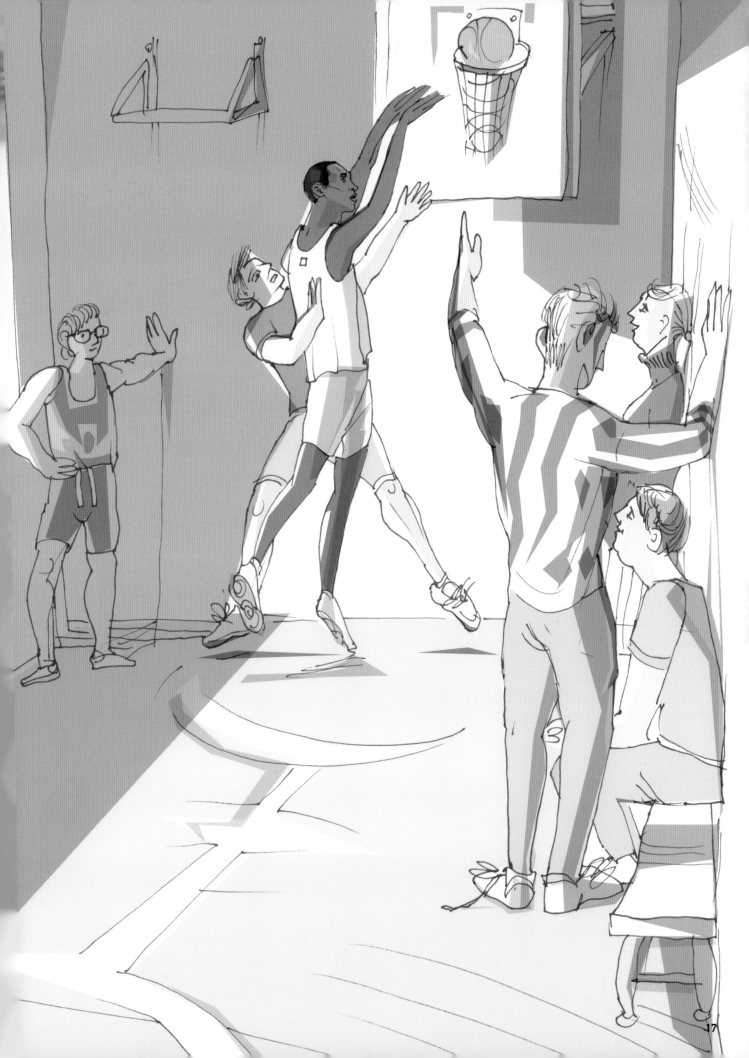

THE PRODIGY

Word of the tall, talented eighth grader soon spread beyond the halls of Bala Cynwyd Middle School and reached the ears of Gregg Downer, a young man in his second year as head coach of the Lower Merion High School boys' basketball team. Eager to see for himself what kind of player was headed his way the following year, Downer invited Kobe to attend one of the Aces practices.

That Lower Merion team would finish the season with an impressive record of 20–5 and be considered one of the best squads in suburban Philadelphia. But they couldn't compete with Kobe, who dominated the older, more experienced players from the moment Downer inserted him into a team scrimmage. Downer could scarcely believe his eyes; Kobe was far and away the best player on the court. After five minutes, he turned to his assistant coaches and said, "This kid is a pro."

Four of the five starters from the Aces team graduated that spring, meaning the 1992–93 season—Kobe's freshman year—was going to be a rebuilding year. In December, the *Philadelphia Inquirer* published a boys' basketball preview package. In it, correspondent Jeremy Treatman noted Lower Merion had one player who offered the inexperienced Aces some hope, writing, "Remember this name: Kobe Bryant."

Unsurprisingly, Kobe not only made the varsity team as a freshman but was also a day-one starter. However, even with their now 6'4" prodigy, Lower Merion often found itself overmatched and outgunned. Though Kobe led the team in scoring by averaging 17.1 points per

game, the Aces won only 4 of their 24 contests that year.

In addition to being the team's most talented player, Kobe was its hardest worker. After each practice, either Downer or Joe, who Downer had hired as an assistant, stayed to rebound for Kobe as he fired hundreds of shots from various spots around the court. Losing never sat well with him, and his determination to win motivated him all the more.

With Kobe a year older and an inch taller and having an entire season of varsity basketball under his belt, the Aces were a much-improved team in Kobe's sophomore year. He wound up averaging 22 points per game that year as the Aces went a respectable 16–6. The next year, Kobe led Lower Merion to a Central League championship. But in the second round of the state tournament, Kobe committed a costly turnover in a game that the Aces would eventually lose.

In the locker room afterward he broke down in tears, apologizing to his teammates for not doing more. He had averaged 31.1 points and 10.4 rebounds per game during his junior season, but in Kobe's mind it wasn't enough. He wanted a state championship and he had just one more crack at it. There was still more work to be done.

1992–96: Kobe shines as Lower Merion's star player. Though he endures some setbacks, he's still determined to win the state championship.

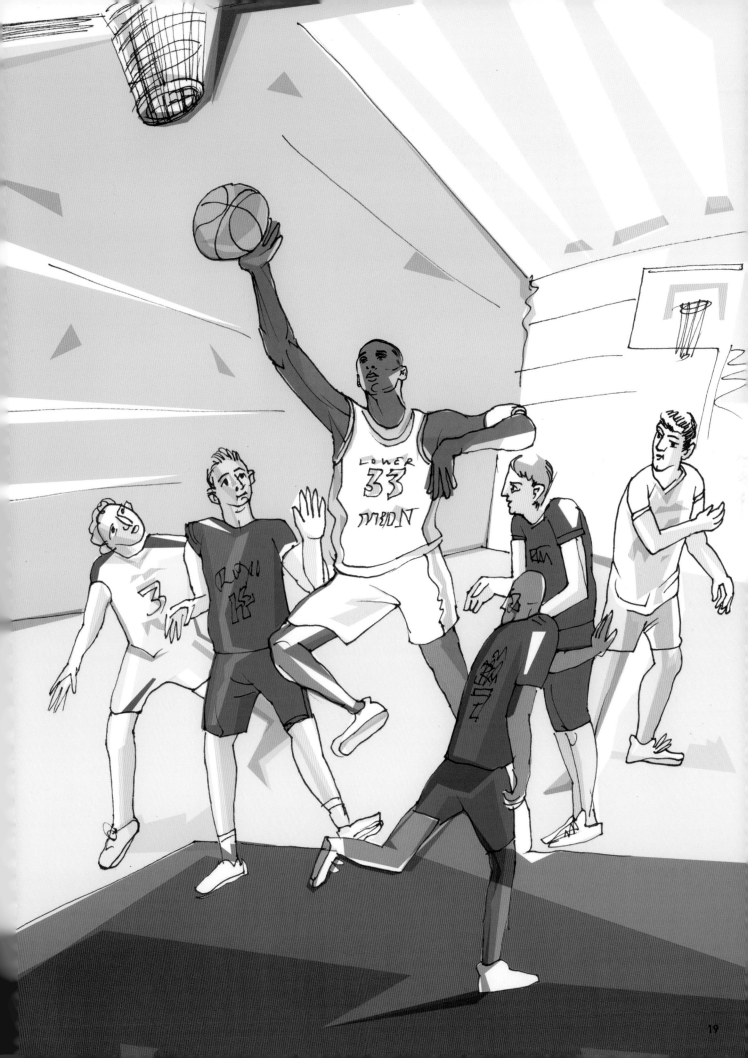

THE SECRET

As Kobe prepared to enter his senior year at Lower Merion, speculation grew about what the prodigy would do beyond high school. Ranked as one of the top prospects in the nation, just about every college in the country vied for his services. But Kobe harbored a secret he had shared with just a few select people: He had no intention of going to college at all. He wanted to turn professional straight out of high school.

The idea of going prep-to-pro was not unprecedented. In fact, that very summer, the Minnesota Timberwolves had selected high school superstar Kevin Garnett with the fifth pick of the 1995 NBA draft. A few other players had also made such a leap, but so far, every high school player drafted directly to the NBA had been a forward or a center. Kobe played the guard position, and no guard had ever attempted such a feat.

History didn't deter Kobe. If anything, it made him all the more determined. And, in the summer of 1995, Kobe got the chance to prove he was ready to compete with the men of the NBA.

One of Kobe's classmates at Lower Merion was Tarvia Lucas, whose father, John, happened to be the head coach of the Philadelphia 76ers. Tarvia told her father he had to come see Kobe play, and so he did. What he saw so impressed him that he invited Kobe to the gym at St. Joseph's College, where many of the 76ers and other NBA players worked out.

Many high school players—even the most talented ones—would be nervous and intimidated by the prospect of scrimmaging against NBA players. Kobe, though, was not like most high schoolers, and he never got scared on the basketball court. In fact, the thought of going up against the game's best only excited him, and he played the same aggressive, attacking brand of basketball he always did. His pure audacity impressed the professionals.

One of those players was 6'10" Rick Mahorn, then of the New Jersey Nets. Mahorn was known for his physical play and had won an NBA title as a member of the Detroit Pistons "Bad Boys" in 1989. When Kobe got the chance, he attempted to "posterize" Mahorn by dunking on him. Mahorn rejected the shot but was amazed Kobe had the gall to even try. "After a while, it kind of popped into my mind that I can play with these guys," Kobe said.

When Kobe wasn't holding his own against professionals, he was dominating his peers. At the ABCD Camp, a prestigious showcase of the top high school players, Kobe won MVP. At the similar Adidas Big Time Tournament, he earned first-team honors. No one doubted Kobe had NBA-level talent, but few people believed the kid would actually forego college.

The time to reveal his secret to the world would come. But first, Kobe had some unfinished business with the Aces to attend to.

1995: Determined to prove himself to the NBA, Kobe trains with star player Rick Mahorn.

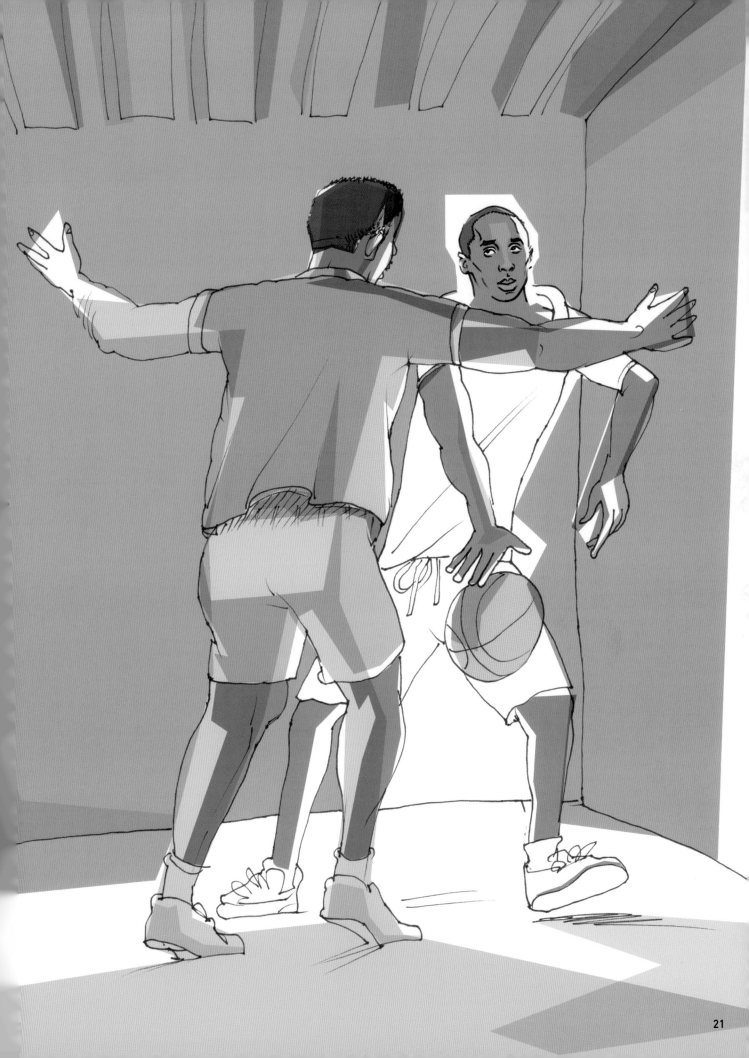

OUT ON TOP

From 1941 to 1943, Lower Merion won three consecutive state championships. Fast-forward to the 1995–96 season, and the program was still in search of its next title. Kobe, now a senior, was determined to end the drought.

To prepare his team for the gauntlet of the state tournament, head coach Gregg Downer purposefully scheduled games with several tough, non-conference teams to begin the season, and the Aces stumbled out of the gate. Playing in a renowned tournament in Myrtle Beach, South Carolina, Lower Merion lost to Jenks (Oklahoma) High School, dropping its record to a pedestrian 4–3.

Downer's team was in trouble. When Kobe was on the bench, the rest of the Aces didn't have the talent to win consistently. However, when Kobe was on the court, his teammates deferred to him so much that Lower Merion might as well have been playing one-on-five. Downer could sense the season slipping away.

Immediately following the Jenks game, Downer called for a team meeting. He turned to each player, telling them exactly what was expected of them. Downer implored Kobe to trust his teammates, reminding his superstar that his job was to make everyone else better. Lower Merion never looked back, winning its final 15 regular season games. As postseason play approached, though, Downer grew increasingly anxious. "Relax, coach," Kobe would say. "I got this."

As it turned out, Downer had nothing to worry about. In Pennsylvania, the postseason consisted of a district tournament, which decided who would qualify for the state tournament. In the District One championship game, Lower Merion faced Chester High School's Clippers. The previous year, the Clippers had humiliated the Aces by 27 points. This time, the Aces went on to win by 60–53, with Kobe chalking up 34 points, 11 rebounds, 6 assists, and 9 blocks. It was on to state.

Lower Merion marched its way to the semifinals of the state tournament, where Chester once again awaited them. With the game tied in overtime, Kobe drilled a shot and then made two free throws to give the Aces a four-point lead. Then, in the final seconds, he zoomed down the court past Chester's entire team and threw down a monstrous slam to seal the game. He ended with 39 points.

The Aces' final opponent, Erie Cathedral Prep's Ramblers, played a slow-paced, deliberate style of basketball. At the half, Lower Merion was down 21–15. With Erie's defense focused entirely on Kobe, it was time for his teammates to step up. In the third quarter, Lower Merion went on an 11–0 run, with Kobe scoring only two of them. Clinging to a two-point lead in the final seconds, Kobe found himself with the ball, swarmed by the Ramblers' defense. Instead of forcing the issue, the superstar slung a pass to one of his teammates, who laid it in, putting the game out of reach. The final whistle blew. The Ramblers had held Kobe to just 17 points, but the Aces had learned to trust each other. Finally, Kobe was a champion.

March 23, 1996: Kobe and his Lower Merion teammates celebrate winning the state championship.

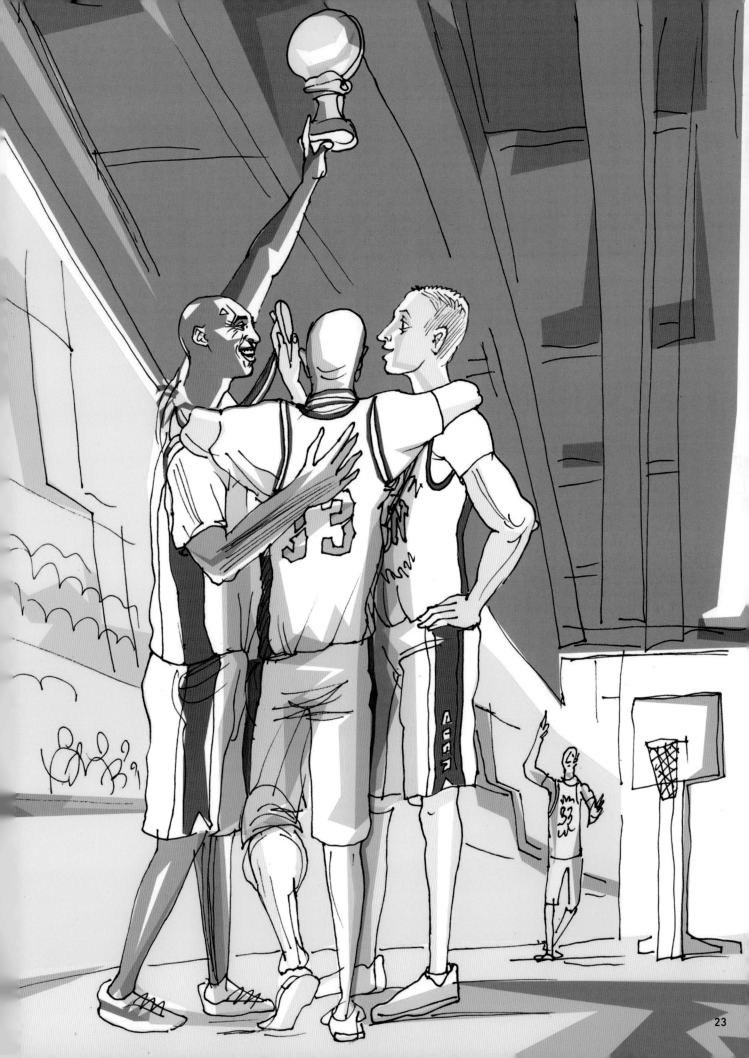

THE DECISION

Throughout his senior year, Kobe kept quiet about his future plans. Rumors spread that the phenom was considering declaring for the NBA draft right out of high school, but when pressed on this by the media, Kobe remained coy, saying he hadn't made up his mind.

Certainly, Kobe had dominated the prep ranks like few before him. During his time at Lower Merion, Kobe amassed a whopping 2,883 points. He also received just about every accolade a high school player can hope for. Following his senior season, Kobe was the Pennsylvania State Player of the Year, a Parade All-American, and a McDonald's All-American. Most impressively, he won the Naismith Award, which is given to the best high school basketball player in the country.

Dominating teenagers on the court is one thing, but doing the same against grown men is quite another. The consensus among scouts and basketball analysts was that the kid should go to college. The college basketball experience was paramount to a player's long-term development and maturity, so the thinking went. Besides, at 6'6", some scouts believed Kobe lacked the size to play forward and didn't yet have the ballhandling or shooting skills to play guard. And even if he had the talent, at 17 years old, could he handle the NBA lifestyle, both from a physical and a mental perspective?

Still, there were some who thought Kobe should make the leap. He could injure himself or underperform in college and damage his NBA prospects. If he had the chance to turn professional now, why wait?

Should Kobe decide to go the college route, he certainly didn't have a lack of options. Among those most vigorously pursuing him was none other than Duke head coach Mike Krzyzewski. "Coach K" had recently won two NCAA national championships with an All-American named Grant Hill, and the legendary coach thought he could do more of the same with Kobe.

As he pondered his future, Kobe had the benefit of having a father who had played in the NBA. Father and son spent hours discussing Kobe's options, but Joe was careful not to push his son one way or another. The choice had to be Kobe's alone.

Kobe announced he would hold a press conference on April 29, 1996, in the gym at Lower Merion after school. His classmates joined the faculty and hundreds of media members to hear his decision. Dressed in a beige silk suit, brown silk tie, and white shirt, with a pair of sunglasses sitting atop his forehead, Kobe confidently strode up to the lectern, paused for dramatic effect, and, with a giant smile across his face, announced, "I have decided to skip college and take my talent to the NBA."

April 29, 1996: At the Lower Merion High School gym, Kobe announces that he's decided to skip college and declare for the NBA draft.

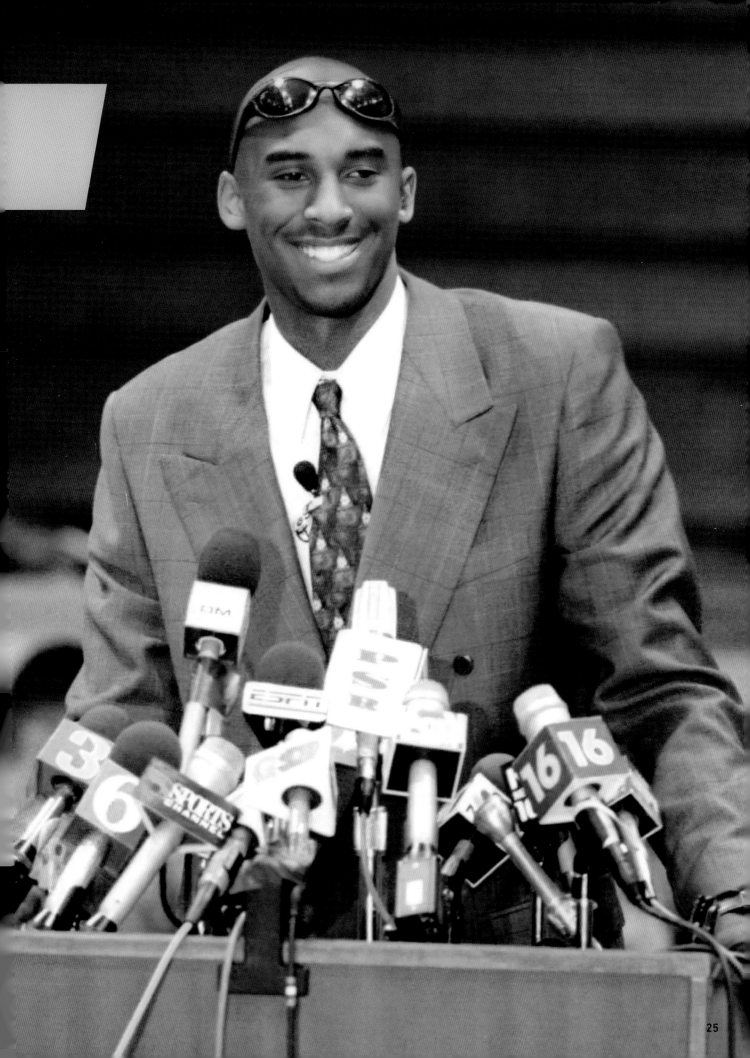

CELEBRITY

Even before he declared his eligibility for the NBA draft, Kobe Bryant's reputation was well known. One evening during his senior year, Philadelphia 76ers' coach John Lucas invited Kobe to a game against the Chicago Bulls. While in Philadelphia's locker room before the game, Lucas asked Kobe if he wanted to meet Michael Jordan. Kobe eagerly agreed.

To the young man's shock and amazement, when Jordan spotted him, he said, "Kobe, what's up?" Kobe had no clue Jordan knew who he was. Jordan then engaged Kobe in conversation, advising him not to become so distracted by the pressure and the hype that the game of basketball became unenjoyable.

After he declared for the draft, though, Kobe reached full-blown celebrity status. His decision became a national story, as every pundit and analyst wanted to provide their take on the situation. Moreover, now that Kobe intended to turn professional, he could start making money from his name. Less than a month following his announcement, Kobe signed a shoe deal with Adidas worth a reported $10 million. In the blink of an eye, the 17-year-old was a multimillionaire.

Any doubts about Kobe's newly minted celebrity status were erased the night of Lower Merion's prom. The press lined up outside the Bellevue Hotel in Philadelphia to await the arrival, in a white limousine, of Kobe and his date, Brandy Norwood. Brandy was a 17-year-old actress and singer who starred in a sitcom called *Moesha* and whose debut album, released in 1994, sold six million copies.

The two had met the night of the 1996 Essence Awards at Madison Square Garden in New York City. Kobe was a guest of Mike Harris, a marketing manager and promoter whose clientele included the R&B vocal group Boyz II Men. Harris, looking to branch out into basketball, befriended Kobe and learned of his crush on Brandy. So, after the awards show, Harris set up a meeting between the two young stars.

In truth, the prom date was as much a public relations ploy as it was a true date. Even so, the two connected over their shared celebrity at such a young age. Brandy had been in the public eye since the age of 14 and so understood better than any of Kobe's high school peers what was awaiting Kobe as he transitioned from high school star to NBA star.

In June, Kobe graduated from Lower Merion. In the 1996 yearbook, Kobe was voted the male student "Most Likely to Succeed." It is likely, however, that even his classmates didn't know just how right they were.

May 25, 1996: Kobe attends his high school prom with Brandy Norwood, a famous singer and actress.

STATUS

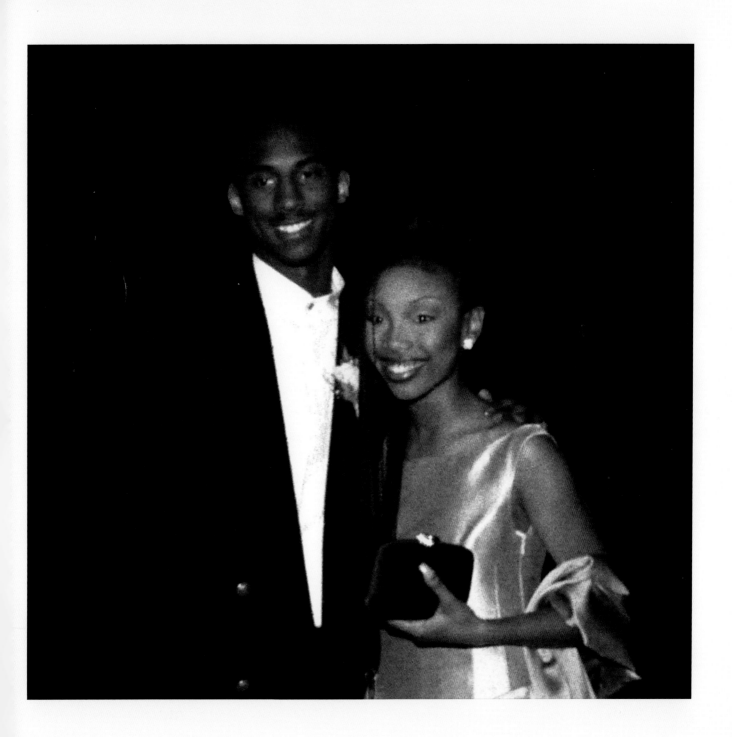

CAREER PREP

NBA franchises were split on their opinions of Kobe heading into the 1996 draft. Kobe was not completely unknown to NBA scouts, some of whom had attended Lower Merion games to see the budding superstar for themselves. Some scouts lauded the teenager's maturity and high basketball IQ, traits perhaps unsurprising for the son of an NBA player who spent his whole life analyzing the game.

Still others couldn't get past Kobe's young age and relative inexperience. They didn't think his skills were NBA-ready, nor did they believe his body could handle the rigors of an 82-game NBA season. Because of these mitigating factors, Kobe was projected to be picked in the middle to later part of the first round of the draft.

Kobe, of course, was not standing by idly in the weeks leading up to the draft. He hired a personal trainer to help strengthen his body. Plus, Joe Bryant asked his friend Tony DiLeo, a former professional player in Europe who at the time was the director of scouting for the 76ers, to prepare Kobe for the pre-draft workouts he would eventually have with select teams.

DiLeo and Bryant would meet each day in the Fieldhouse at St. Joseph's University, with DiLeo having Kobe run a drill that required him to shoot 300 shots from various spots on the floor. The catch was, should Kobe miss three straight shots from any one spot, he would have to start the drill over again. "That's when I saw this inner drive he had," DiLeo said. "He was relentless."

A handful of teams showed interest in Kobe. Among them were the New Jersey Nets, Boston Celtics, and Phoenix Suns. Two teams, though, intrigued Kobe more than the rest: his hometown 76ers and the Los Angeles Lakers.

The 76ers held the No. 1 overall pick, and though there were some in the organization, DiLeo included, who pushed management to select the hometown hero, it was never likely the team would gamble the No. 1 pick on a high schooler.

The Lakers, meanwhile, held the 24th pick. Even the most pessimistic projections didn't have Kobe falling that far. If Los Angeles was serious about acquiring Kobe, they would have to find a way to move up in the draft. It just so happened that the Lakers general manager, Jerry West, a Hall of Fame player and NBA legend, was serious about making Kobe a Laker. And he was already formulating a plan to get him.

November 25, 1996: Kobe looks to score during his rookie season with the Lakers. He worked hard to make his first season a success, but there were still challenges to overcome.

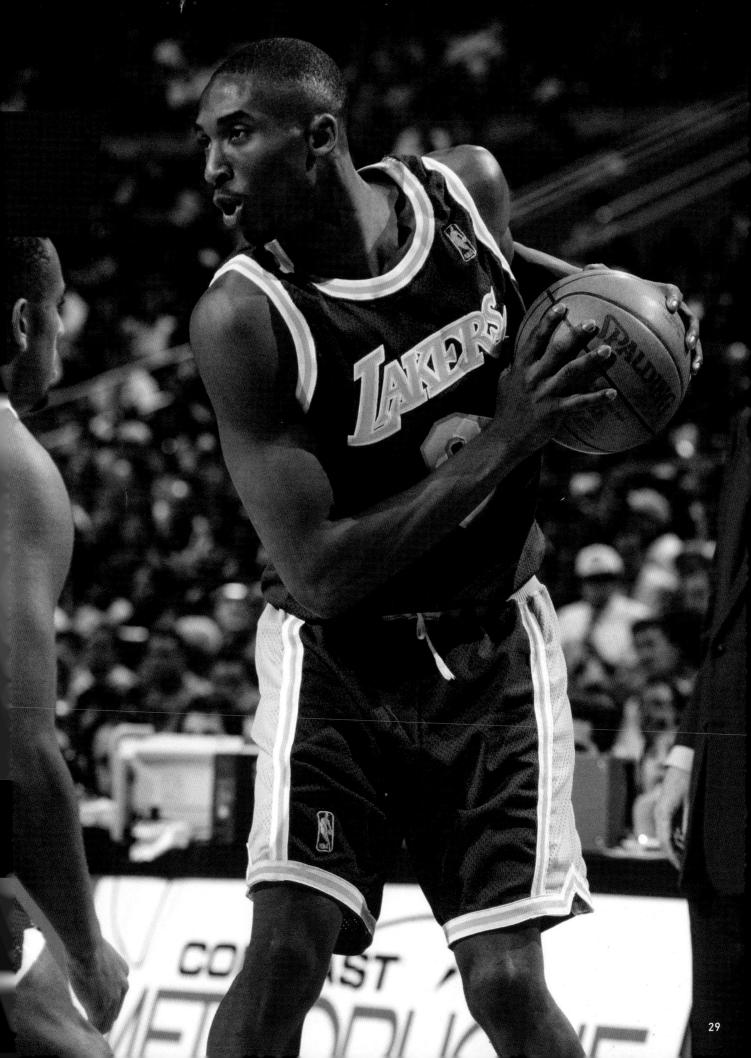

JERRY'S

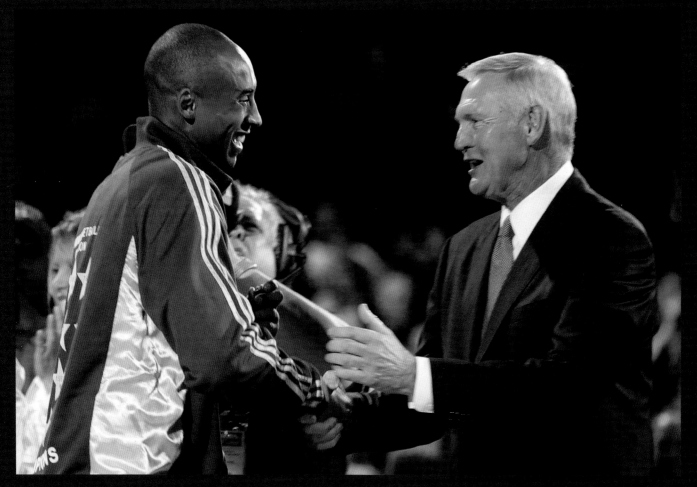

October 27, 2009: Jerry West's hunch about Bryant proves right—here he is congratulating the NBA champion.

In his playing days from 1960–74, Jerry West led the Lakers to the NBA Finals nine times, though they won only once. Standing 6'4", West was known for his all-around talent and ability to perform well in high-pressure situations. He earned a reputation for being someone who would do anything to win.

In the summer of 1996, now as Los Angeles's general manager, West was trying to rebuild a Lakers franchise that had run into some tough times after Magic Johnson had led them to five titles in the 1980s. West was intrigued by Kobe,

who reminded West of himself. So even though the Lakers wouldn't pick until well after Kobe was expected to be drafted, West arranged a workout for Kobe.

During the session, West asked Kobe to go one-on-one against Lakers assistant coach Michael Cooper. Now 40, Cooper was known as one of the best perimeter defenders in the NBA during his playing years, and he kept himself in great shape. West was stunned by the way Kobe relentlessly attacked the basket when he had the ball and the way he challenged Cooper on defense.

VISION

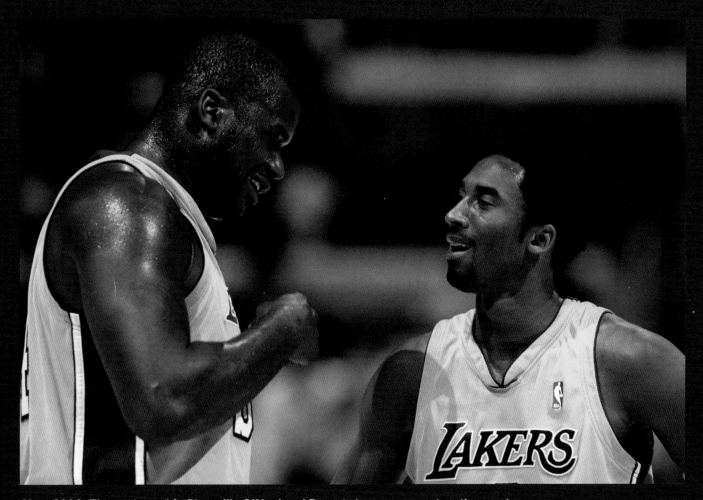

Circa 2000: The unstoppable Shaquille O'Neal and Bryant share a moment on the court.

After 15 minutes, West stopped the work-out. He had seen everything he needed to see. "[Kobe] was the most skilled player we've ever worked out, the kind of skill you don't see very often," West said later. He decided he would do whatever it took to acquire the teenager.

But Kobe was just part one of West's two-pronged plan to restore the Lakers to their former glory. He also had his eye on prized free agent center Shaquille O'Neal, who had spent his first four years playing for the Orlando

Magic. The Lakers' dynasty of the 1980s was built around Johnson and center Kareem Abdul-Jabbar, and West envisioned recreating that magic with Kobe and Shaq.

To make this dream a reality, West had his work cut out for him. Not only did he have to outbid every other team for O'Neal's services, but he also had to find a way to trade up in the draft. And that required a trading partner. But what team would be willing to do business with Jerry West and the Los Angeles Lakers?

DRAFT NIGHT

Vlade Divac had spent all seven seasons of his NBA career with the Los Angeles Lakers, who drafted the Serbian center in the first round of the 1989 draft. He had developed into a solid player for the Lakers, averaging 16 points and 10.4 rebounds per game during the 1994–95 season. But he was no Shaquille O'Neal. And with Jerry West's eyes set on O'Neal, Divac became expendable.

In the days leading up to the 1996 NBA draft, West desperately sought a way to trade up in a bid to draft Kobe. He first called the New Jersey Nets, offering them Divac in exchange for the eighth pick of the evening. The Nets rebuffed West. They had already decided who they wanted to take with their pick: Kobe Bryant.

But Kobe preferred to play for Los Angeles, and he made his desire clear to New Jersey's management, going so far as threatening to leave the NBA to play professionally in Europe if the Nets drafted him. Some in the Nets organization were willing to call Kobe's bluff. But New Jersey's young head coach, John Calipari, started having second thoughts and decided they would draft Villanova star Kerry Kittles if he was available.

The Nets were seemingly no longer a draft threat to Kobe, but West still needed a trading partner, and he finally found one in the Charlotte Hornets. Already possessing a star forward named Glen Rice, Charlotte's management believed they were one center away from becoming contenders. They wanted Divac. So Charlotte and Los Angeles made an agreement in principle: If Kobe was available when the Hornets picked 13th, they would draft Kobe and then trade him to Los Angeles for Divac.

West entered the night of June 26 cautiously optimistic he would come away with his No. 1 target, but draft night was always unpredictable, and it was far from certain that things would shake out the way he wanted. As expected, Philadelphia kicked things off by drafting Georgetown guard Allen Iverson. The next six teams all passed on Kittles, who, just as Calipari had planned, the Nets grabbed at No. 8.

Five picks later, Charlotte selected Kobe. Everything had gone exactly to plan, and Kobe appeared to be on his way to Los Angeles. But then it looked like it would all fall apart. Divac threatened to retire rather than play for Charlotte, and so Charlotte general manager Bob Bass called West to say the deal was off. West assured Bass that Divac would not retire, but Bass was not persuaded. The deal was still in flux several days later until Divac's wife finally convinced her husband not to retire.

On July 1, the teams made the deal official. Kobe was now a Laker. Later that month, West completed his vision, signing Shaquille O'Neal to a seven-year, $120 million contract, the largest contract in league history. Would they bring the title back to Los Angeles?

July 12, 1996: The Lakers introduce their newest member, teenage sensation Kobe Bryant.

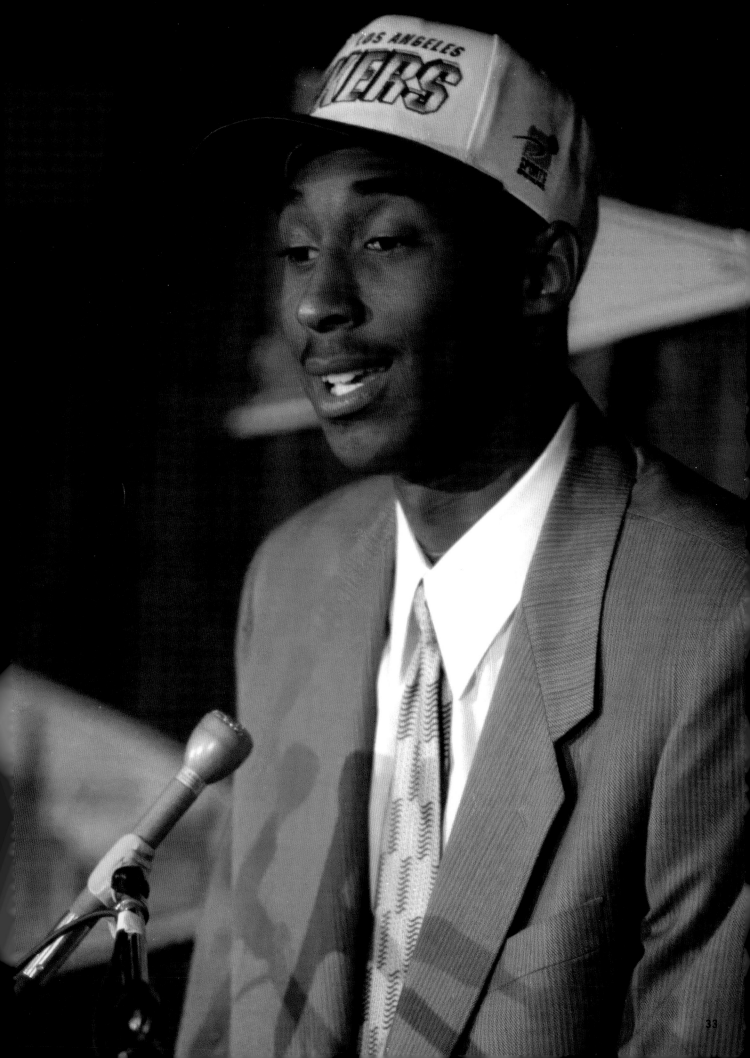

ROOKIE BLUES

In July, Kobe flew to Los Angeles to sign his rookie contract, a three-year deal worth $3.65 million. While waiting for his luggage at the airport, somebody approached him and said, "You must be a basketball player. Who do you play for?" Instinctively, Kobe started to say, "Lower Merion," before catching himself and replying, "I guess I'm a Laker."

He purchased a home nestled on a hillside in the Pacific Palisades. His father, mother, and sister Shaya moved in with him, recognizing the 17-year-old would need a support system he could trust.

Kobe was living his dream, but then the season started. Things began going awry even before training camp opened in October. In September, Kobe was playing in a pick-up game when he fell and cracked a bone in his left wrist, rendering him unable to play when Los Angeles's official practices started.

He also found it difficult to connect with his much older teammates. After practice, many Lakers liked to enjoy Los Angeles's nightlife, but Kobe wasn't old enough to get into the clubs.

Simultaneously drafting Kobe while signing Shaq sent somewhat of a mixed message to the Lakers organization. While Kobe was more of a long-term, developmental project, Shaq didn't join the team to win at some later date. His presence meant the Lakers were supposed to contend now, and contending now didn't necessarily mean giving a teenage rookie a ton of minutes on the court.

To start the season, Lakers coach Del Harris played Kobe only sparingly, usually in the final minutes of games that had long since been decided. Kobe didn't record his first NBA basket until the season's fifth game. Then, after the All-Star break, point guard Nick Van Exel went down with an injury, opening up playing time for the rookie. Kobe played well, proving he could score on the professional level.

By the time the playoffs rolled around, Kobe found his playing time increasing. The Lakers defeated the Portland Trailblazers in the first round, with Kobe even scoring 22 points in Game 3 of that series. The Utah Jazz were the Lakers' next opponent, and Utah jumped out to a commanding 3–1 series lead, meaning Los Angeles had to win the next game to keep their season alive.

With the score tied in the closing seconds of Game 5 and O'Neal having fouled out, Harris decided to put the game in his rookie's hands, telling his team to get Kobe the ball and get out of his way. Kobe made a move on his defender, pulled up from about 14 feet, and launched . . . an airball. The game went into overtime, during which Kobe shot three more airballs. The Jazz won, and Kobe walked off the court humbled and humiliated—but not defeated.

On the flight home, Kobe called his agent's assistant and told her to make sure the local high school gym was open when he landed. It was past 10 p.m. local time, but the assistant made some calls. The gym would be open.

The plane landed at 2 a.m., and Kobe drove directly to the high school. He stayed until sunrise, shooting shot after shot after shot. Kobe wouldn't let his team down like that ever again.

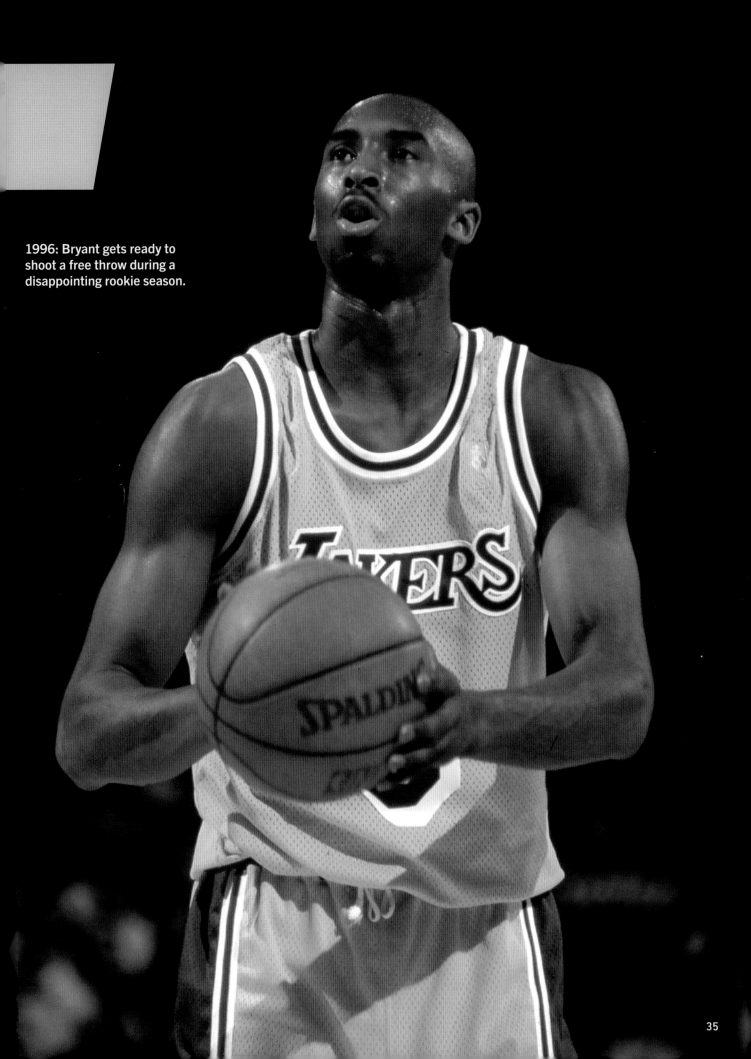

1996: Bryant gets ready to shoot a free throw during a disappointing rookie season.

Kobe spent his first offseason working hard on his game. In addition to spending time in the gym, he incorporated a rigorous weight-training program into his fitness routine in an effort to improve his strength. Ruminating on what had gone wrong at the end of regulation during that final game against Utah, Kobe concluded he had shot the airball in a moment of indecision. He had intended to drive all the way to the basket but pulled up for a jumper instead.

Kobe vowed never to second-guess himself again. If he saw an opportunity to attack, he would, regardless of who may be waiting for him at the basket. He would never again talk himself out of doing the one thing that came most naturally to him.

As the 1997–98 season began, Coach Harris once again relegated Kobe to the bench. But his role had expanded from the previous year, and Kobe was often the first substitute to enter a game. Also, because Kobe played on Los Angeles's second unit, he was often on the floor while Shaq was resting, which allowed him to become the focal point of the Lakers' offense. Kobe was tasked with bringing energy off the bench and putting the ball in the hoop.

Kobe excelled in this role. The Lakers won their first 11 games, and Kobe averaged almost 20 points per game during this stretch—an incredible figure for a bench player. Moreover, he was quickly becoming one of the most exciting—and popular—players in the game. This was confirmed when the fans voted Kobe onto the All-Star

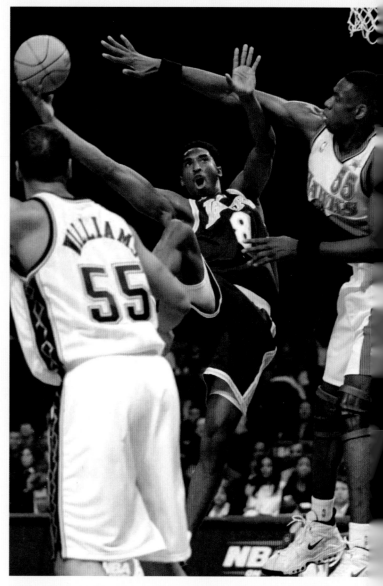

February 8, 1998: At the All-Star Game, Bryant prepares to score past Hawks' player Dikembe Mutumbo.

team. In fact, Kobe garnered more votes than any other player, even Michael Jordan.

On February 8, 1998, at Madison Square Garden, at the age of 19, Kobe officially became the youngest person to start an NBA All-Star Game. The moment was not too big for the teenager, who led

ALL-STAR

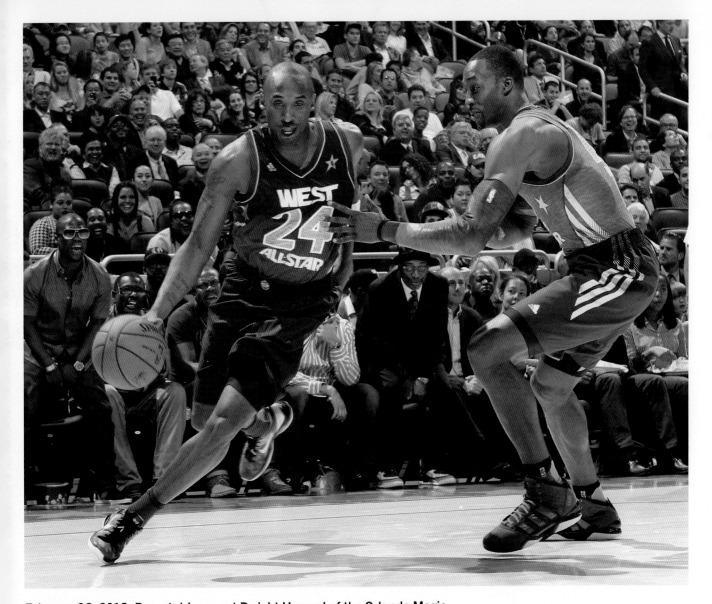

February 26, 2012: Bryant drives past Dwight Howard of the Orlando Magic at the All-Star Game.

the Western Conference squad with 18 points and went toe-to-toe with Jordan. In the end, the veteran would get the best of the upstart, scoring 23 points and securing MVP honors as the East prevailed against the West.

Still, Kobe had proved he belonged with the league's very best. From that year forward, he made every possible All-Star team and won four All-Star MVP Awards. In his 20-year career, the only two seasons he wasn't an All-Star were his rookie season and in 1999, when the game was canceled because of a lockout.

THE PAYOFF

Though the Lakers finished tied with the second-best record in the Western Conference in 1998, they fell short in the playoffs. Once again, they were ousted by Utah, this time in the Western Conference Finals in a four-game sweep.

After the loss, Kobe was asked how he intended to spend his offseason. "Basketball," Kobe responded. "That's all." But the 1998–99 season was nothing short of a disaster. The players' union's contract with the owners had expired without a new agreement in place, and in June 1998, the owners responded by "locking out" the players, meaning no team activities could take place.

The lockout didn't end until January 1999, and when play resumed, the Lakers found themselves in disarray. A rift had developed between Kobe and Shaq. The big man felt that Kobe, now a full-time starter, tried to take over too often, while Kobe questioned Shaq's work ethic.

Los Angeles got off to a rocky start, and coach Del Harris was subsequently fired. Interim head coach Kurt Rambis failed to exert control over his team. Management felt more changes were necessary, so All-Star guard Eddie Jones and backup center Elden Campbell were traded to Charlotte for sharpshooter Glen Rice and forward J. R. Reid. In the end, the Lakers were swept out of the playoffs in the second round by the champions, the San Antonio Spurs.

The Kobe-Shaq experiment was now going into its fourth year with virtually nothing to show for it. Jerry West still believed in his star duo, but something was missing. West decided that the missing ingredient wasn't a player at all but the right coach. He persuaded former Chicago coach Phil Jackson to come out of retirement for the 1999–2000 season. Jackson had won six titles with the Jordan-led Bulls and knew how to handle star players with big egos.

The move worked. Kobe and Shaq both thrived in Jackson's famed triangle offense, which relies on spacing and movement to get players open. Kobe's blend of speed and agility was perfectly suited for the triangle, and his game blossomed. Not only did he average 22.5 points per game, he led the team in assists as well.

Jackson had the Lakers firing on all cylinders, and they finished the year with a league-best record of 67–15—a full 11 games better than the next-best team. They marched into the Western Conference Finals, where the Portland Trailblazers pushed them to seven games.

In the deciding seventh game, Kobe and Shaq's newfound chemistry was on full display. After rallying from a 13-point, fourth-quarter deficit, the Lakers clung to a four-point lead with under a minute to play. With the ball at the top of the key, Kobe used a killer crossover to blow past Scottie Pippen and, when the defense collapsed on him, lobbed a beautiful alley-oop pass to Shaq, who slammed it home with one hand, sealing the game for the Lakers.

After three years of disappointment, the Lakers were heading to the finals, with the Indiana Pacers the only thing standing between Kobe and a ring.

2000: A focused Bryant dribbles a ball up the court.

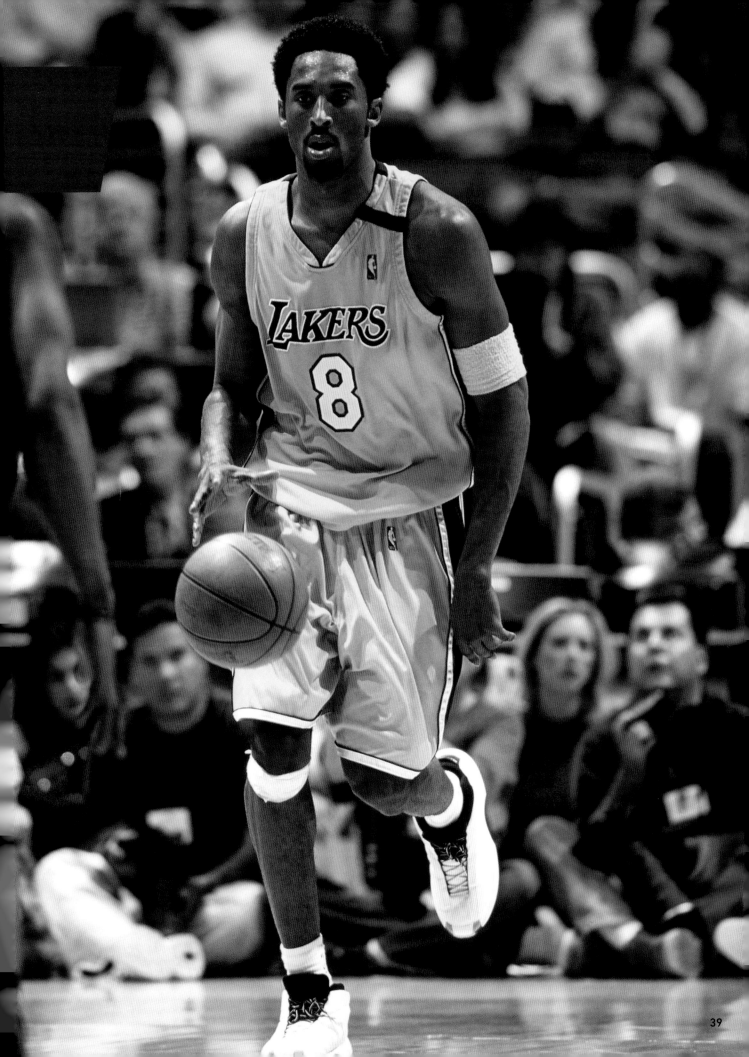

THREEPEAT

The Lakers dominated Game 1 of the 2000 NBA Finals against the Pacers, winning by a score of 104–87. Late in the first quarter of Game 2, though, Bryant suffered a badly sprained ankle. Although Los Angeles held on to win, their star's status for the rest of the series was in doubt.

Bryant missed Game 3, which the Pacers won, and it didn't look like he would be able to suit up for Game 4 either. The Lakers appeared to be in trouble, but right before the game, Bryant decided his ankle felt good enough to play.

The fourth quarter ended in a 104–104 tie, and then early in overtime, O'Neal fouled out. As Shaq walked to the bench, Kobe told him, "Don't worry about it, I got it." Bad ankle and all, Kobe proceeded to hit three clutch shots, including an offensive rebound put-back in the closing seconds as the Lakers squeaked by with a 120–118 victory.

Los Angeles went on to win the series in six games, with Bryant pouring in 26 points in the finale. As the buzzer sounded, Kobe and Shaq hugged each other. Finally, they had proven they could win a championship together.

They were just getting started.

Shaq struggled through some injuries as the Lakers set out to defend their title during the 2000–2001 season. Kobe picked up the slack, earning Player of the Month honors in December after averaging 32.3 points, 4.9 assists, and 4.8 rebounds.

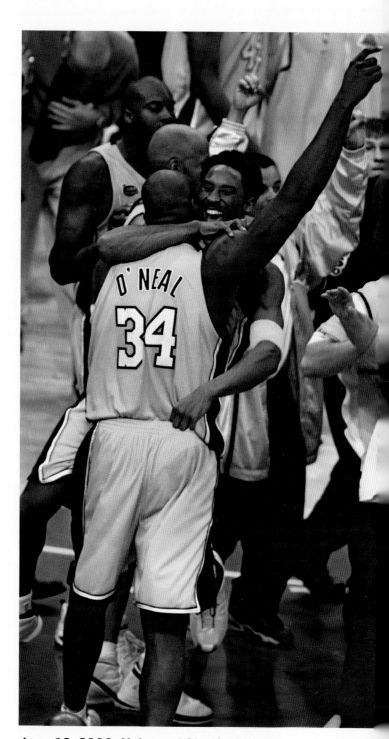

June 19, 2000: Kobe and Shaq celebrate defeating the Indiana Pacers at the NBA Finals—their first championship win.

The Lakers swept all three of their Western Conference opponents before dropping Game 1 of the finals against Allen Iverson's Philadelphia 76ers. It was the only game Los Angeles lost throughout the entire postseason. They won the next four games to capture their second straight championship, finishing the playoffs with an unprecedented record of 15–1.

In 2001–2, Los Angeles looked to keep the party going for a third consecutive season. The Lakers stormed through the regular season, but in the Western Conference Finals they found themselves down 3–2 against old friend Vlade Divac and the Sacramento Kings.

In Game 6, Kobe and Shaq combined for 72 points as the Lakers won a four-point thriller to force a Game 7. The decisive contest went into overtime, when Kobe hit two clutch free throws—his 29th and 30th points of the night—to seal the win for the Lakers. They then breezed through the finals, sweeping the New Jersey Nets in four games.

At the age of 23, Bryant became the youngest player in NBA history to win three championships, and it wasn't lost on anyone that the last team to threepeat was Michael Jordan's Bulls. Kobe and the Lakers were on top of the world. But what goes up must come down, and that 2002 championship would be the last one Kobe and Shaq would win as teammates.

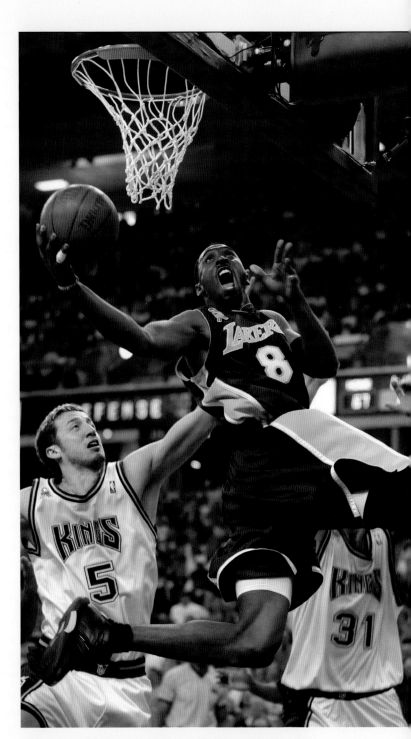

May 18, 2002: During the playoffs, Bryant brings the Lakers to a victory over the Sacramento Kings.

DARK DAYS

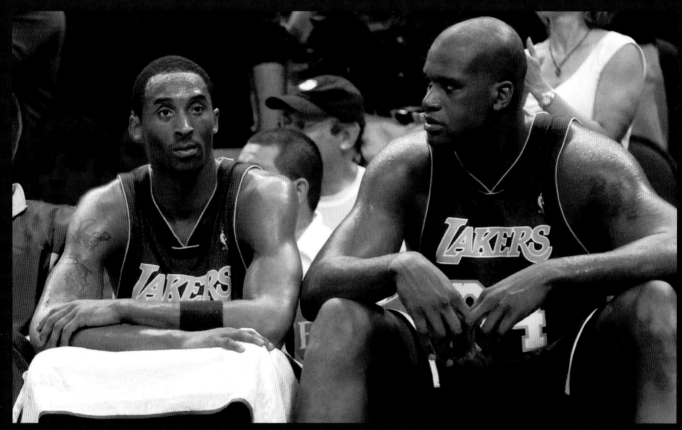

May 2, 2004: A dejected Kobe and Shaq sit on the sidelines as the Lakers lose Game 2 of the Western Conference Semifinals to the San Antonio Spurs.

Kobe's relationship with Shaq began to deteriorate again. O'Neal struggled with a toe injury throughout the 2001–2 season but waited until September 2002 to have surgery, meaning he would miss the start of the 2002–3 season. Bryant thought O'Neal could have addressed the issue earlier in the offseason. The Lakers never quite got rolling and were eliminated in the playoffs by the San Antonio Spurs.

The Lakers tried to retool the next season, but it proved challenging for many reasons. Most gravely, in the 2003 offseason, while Bryant was in Colorado for knee surgery, a young hotel employee accused him of sexual assault, a seri-

ous allegation that threatened Bryant's freedom. This episode negatively affected Bryant's clean-cut image and strained his relationship with his wife, Vanessa, whom he had married in 2001. In 2004, the charges against him were dropped, and Bryant publicly apologized to his accuser.

On the court, the Lakers never fully gelled but nevertheless made it to the NBA Finals against the Detroit Pistons. But while the Pistons played like a well-oiled machine, Bryant and O'Neal seemed out of sync, and Detroit captured the title in five games.

Afterward, the wheels totally fell off. Phil Jackson, who described Bryant as "uncoachable,"

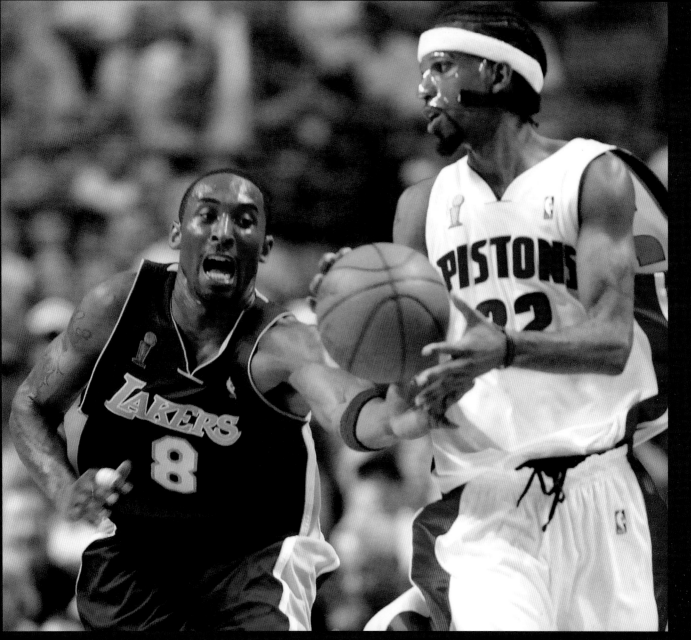

June 15, 2004: During the 2004 NBA Finals, a determined Kobe steals the ball from the Detroit Pistons' Richard Hamilton.

said he wouldn't return if Bryant did. The Lakers prioritized their still-young star, and Jackson retired. Meanwhile, the rift between Kobe and Shaq devolved into an unbridgeable chasm. On July 14, 2004, the Lakers agreed to trade Shaq to the Miami Heat for a trio of players and a draft pick.

After eight seasons of sharing the spotlight with Shaq, the 2004–5 Lakers were indisputably now Bryant's team. He continued to excel individually, but the team struggled to win games, and the Lakers missed the playoffs for the first time since 1994.

That offseason, Kobe mended his relationship with Jackson, and the Lakers rehired the legendary coach. Over the next two seasons, Kobe reached new heights as a scorer. In 2006, he led the league while averaging an astonishing 35.4 points per game, the most scored by any player since Michael Jordan averaged 37.1 in 1987. However, he found team success elusive, as the Lakers were bounced from the playoffs in the first round each of those two seasons. To make matters worse, Shaq had won a championship without Kobe in 2006. Critics were beginning to question whether Kobe would ever be able to do the same without Shaq.

THE BLACK

Amid his off-court struggles in 2003–4, Bryant at some point sat down and watched a movie called *Kill Bill*, directed by Quentin Tarantino. In one scene, an assassin uses a snake known as a black mamba to kill another character. Intrigued by the animal, Bryant did some research on the highly venomous snake and learned it had a 99 percent striking accuracy at high speeds and in quick succession. That was just the type of surgical precision Bryant wanted in his game.

At the same time, he felt his life was spiraling out of control. The court case against him was taking its toll; his family was on the verge of collapsing. "I went from a person who was at the top of his game, had everything coming, to a year later, having absolutely no idea where life is going or if you are even going to be a part of life as we all know it," Bryant said.

He felt the need to separate his personal life from his professional one, and so he decided to create an alter ego. "Kobe" would handle the personal stuff. But from now on, "the Black Mamba" would handle business on the basketball court.

Once he adopted the Black Mamba persona, Bryant felt free to unleash all of his frustrations onto his basketball opponents. Every time he stepped onto the court—whether for practice or a

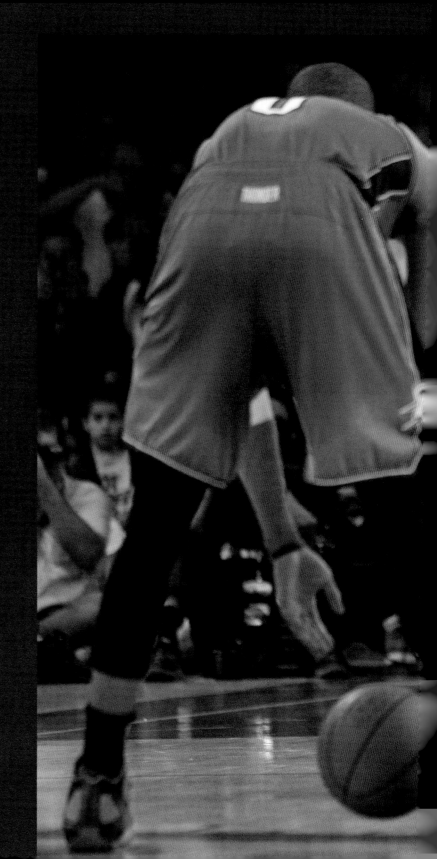

MAMBA

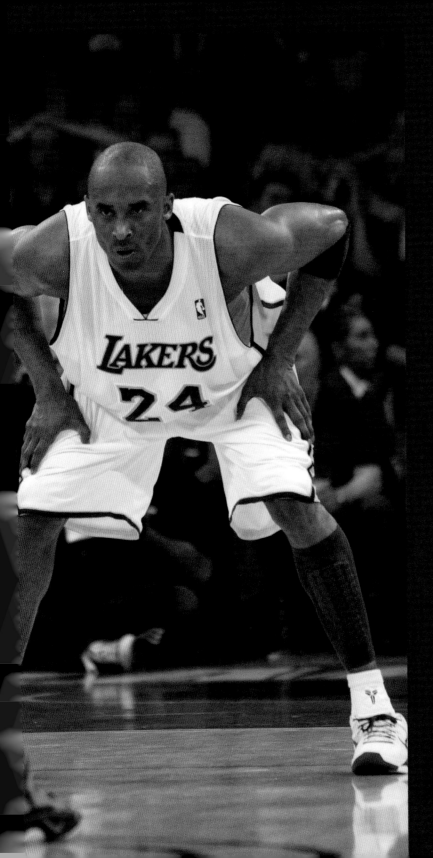

game—he became a stone-cold killer who used his speed, strength, and athleticism to destroy anyone who got in his way.

Over time, the nickname evolved into more of an outlook, something Bryant called "the Black Mamba Mentality." To Bryant, this meant doing whatever it took to overcome obstacles in order to reach his goals. As Bryant entered the second stage of his career—the stage that followed the Colorado incident and the breaking up of the Kobe-Shaq dynasty—it was the Mamba Mentality that fueled him, that drove him to prove his critics wrong.

The Mamba Mentality meant "staying in the moment" and "falling in love with the journey." It meant striving for perfection and greatness. It soon became synonymous with Kobe's unrelenting passion and drive to succeed. It was a mentality his teammates learned to adopt as well, perhaps as the only way to coexist with their determined—and demanding—teammate.

And it meant trouble for the rest of the NBA. For the Black Mamba was angry, and, when provoked, black mambas are deadly dangerous.

April 22, 2012: The driven Black Mamba meets Russell Westbrook of the Oklahoma City Thunder.

81

In the 2005–6 season, Bryant routinely scored more than 30—or even 40—points per game. In fact, on December 20, 2005, against the Dallas Mavericks, the All-NBA shooting guard dropped a career-high 62 points in the Lakers' 112–90 victory.

So when Bryant walked off the court with 26 points at halftime of Los Angeles's game against the Toronto Raptors on January 22, 2006, it seemed like business as usual. The Lakers began the third quarter down 14, a deficit that ballooned to 18 a couple of minutes into the period. Then, the Black Mamba took over.

With 10:42 left in the quarter, Bryant drove to the basket and made a layup. It began a remarkable stretch that saw him make eight shots in a row, including four three-pointers. Bryant's brilliance was on full display, and the Lakers clawed their way back into the game. Bryant's dunk with 1:10 remaining in the third gave the Lakers an 87–85 lead. Los Angeles ended the quarter up six, marking a 20-point turnaround. For the quarter, Kobe scored 27 points on 11–15 shooting.

Bryant already had 53 points and there was still a whole quarter left. The crowd brimmed with anticipation, understanding they were witnessing something historic. In the final 12 minutes, Kobe kept scoring at a relentless pace, hitting jumpers and threes and drawing fouls by attacking the rim with abandon.

His three-pointer with 4:52 remaining put him at 70 points. He hit two more field goals and knocked down five additional free throws, putting him at 79 points with under a minute to go. The crowd began to chant; they wanted their hero to reach 80. Then, with 43.4 seconds remaining, Bryant drew yet another foul. He stepped to the free throw line, and with his fans chanting "M-V-P, M-V-P," he sank them both, giving him 81 for the night.

The Lakers won the game 122–104, but the outcome was almost immaterial compared to Bryant's performance. He made 28 of his 46 shot attempts, including seven threes, and hit 18 of 20 free throws. In the second half alone, Bryant dropped 55 points. The Raptors team scored just 41 during the same period. "I've seen some remarkable games, but I've never seen one like that before," said Phil Jackson, who had coached Michael Jordan during his prime.

Kobe's 81 points are still the second-highest in a single game in NBA history, behind only Wilt Chamberlain's 100 on March 2, 1962. "It turned into something special," Bryant said after his historic performance. "To sit here and say I grasp what happened, that would be lying."

January 22, 2006: Kobe drives to the basket and ultimately scores 81 points in a game against the Toronto Raptors.

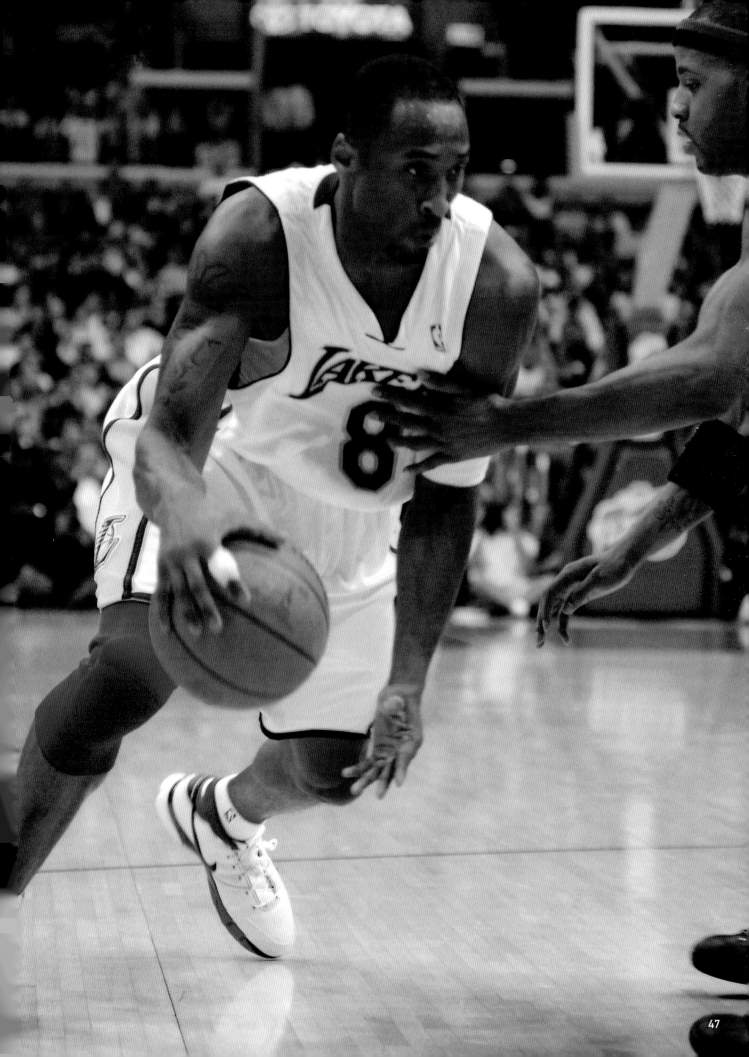

REDEEM TEAM

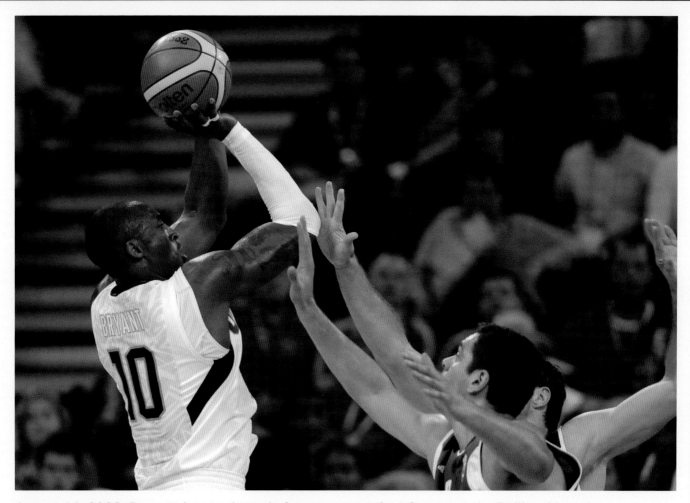

August 14, 2008: Bryant aims to shoot during a game against Greece at the Beijing Olympics.

After losing to the Phoenix Suns in the opening round of the 2007 playoffs, Bryant's frustration with the Lakers organization reached a boiling point. During a radio interview, Bryant upended basketball's offseason by requesting a trade.

Several teams expressed interest, chief among them the Chicago Bulls and Los Angeles Clippers. After a few weeks of wild speculation, Bryant met with Lakers head coach Phil Jackson. It is unclear what the two discussed, but afterward Bryant rescinded his trade demand.

The Lakers played well at the start of the 2007–8 season, and management decided to swing for the fences. On February 1, 2008, the Lakers traded a slew of role players for Memphis Grizzlies All-Star Pau Gasol. Gasol fit in well, and Los Angeles earned the top seed in the Western Conference. Bryant, who won his first and only MVP Award that season, finally led his team to the NBA Finals. However, the Lakers lost to the Boston Celtics in six games.

Bryant had no time to dwell on the disappointment. He had been selected to represent Team USA at the 2008 Beijing Olympics. An injury had kept him off the 2004 squad that failed to win a gold medal for the first time since NBA players

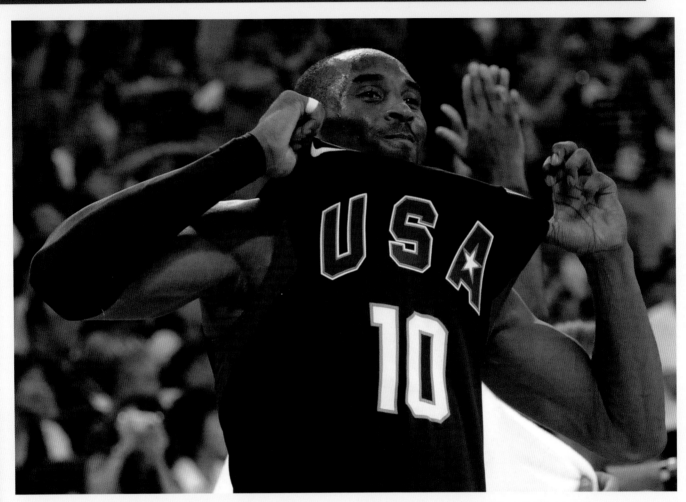

August 24, 2008: Kobe celebrates winning gold at the Beijing Olympics.

began participating in the Olympics, in 1992. The embarrassment of finishing with a bronze medal led to changes in the way Team USA operated. Among those changes, USA Basketball appointed Duke University's Mike Krzyzewski as its head coach.

The pressure on Team USA to reclaim gold was enormous, but critics thought Bryant's "me first" attitude would harm the team's chances. Instead, Bryant set the standard for hard work and selflessness. Before the start of competition, Bryant had visited Krzyzewski's office and told him he wanted the responsibility

of guarding the opposing team's best player.

During the games, the Mamba Mentality was on full display. In a group play victory over the Spanish team (led by Pau Gasol), Bryant knocked his Lakers teammate to the floor when Gasol tried to set a pick on Bryant. In the rematch against Spain for the gold medal, Kobe poured in 13 fourth-quarter points, including a crucial four-point play, to squash a late rally by the Spaniards.

Team USA earned its "Redeem Team" moniker by capturing gold. Perhaps just as important, Bryant used the experience to grow as a player, a teammate, and a leader.

BACK ON TOP

Kobe looked to carry the momentum from Beijing into the 2008–9 NBA season. The Lakers quickly proved they were a force to be reckoned with, winning their first 7 games and 21 out of their first 24 contests. With Bryant as the leader, Los Angeles displayed genuine chemistry—both on and off the court.

That season, Bryant blossomed into one of the best all-around players in the NBA. No longer did Los Angeles need to rely solely on Bryant at all times, but on any given night he was capable of turning in an amazing individual performance. For example, in a February game against the New York Knicks, Bryant scored 61 points, the most ever in Madison Square Garden's storied history.

The Lakers finished the season with a record of 65–17 and returned to the finals after dispatching the Denver Nuggets in the penultimate round. Awaiting them were the upstart Orlando Magic; Kobe averaged 32.4 points and 7.4 assists per game as the Lakers beat the Magic in five games.

At last, seven years after winning his third title, Bryant had a fourth. This time, he had done it as the bona fide alpha. For the first time, Bryant was named the Finals MVP.

The next season, the Lakers reached the finals for the third consecutive year. This time, Bryant would have a chance at sweet revenge, as their opponent once again was the Boston Celtics. Los Angeles lost Games 4 and 5 in Boston, digging themselves into a 3–2 hole, one loss away from defeat. In the locker room after the Game 5 loss, the team looked dejected. Out of nowhere, Bryant stunned his teammates when he started laughing. Bewildered, they asked him what was so funny. "If we started the season and they told us that all we had to go do was go home and win

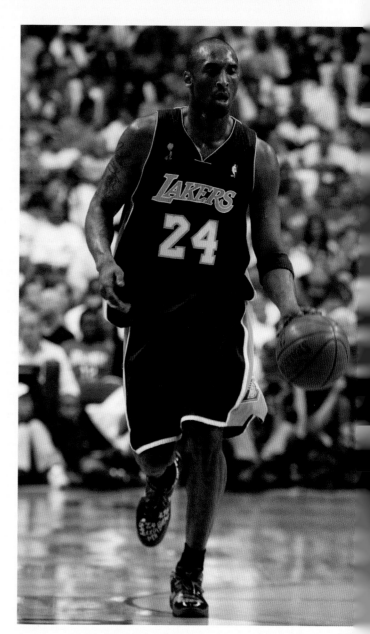

June 14, 2009: Bryant at Game 5 of the NBA Finals— the Lakers win against the Orlando Magic.

two games to be NBA champions, would you take that deal?" They would. In Game 6, the Lakers rolled to an 89–67 win, setting up a winner-take-all Game 7.

In that decisive game, Boston opened up a 13-point third-quarter lead before the Lakers

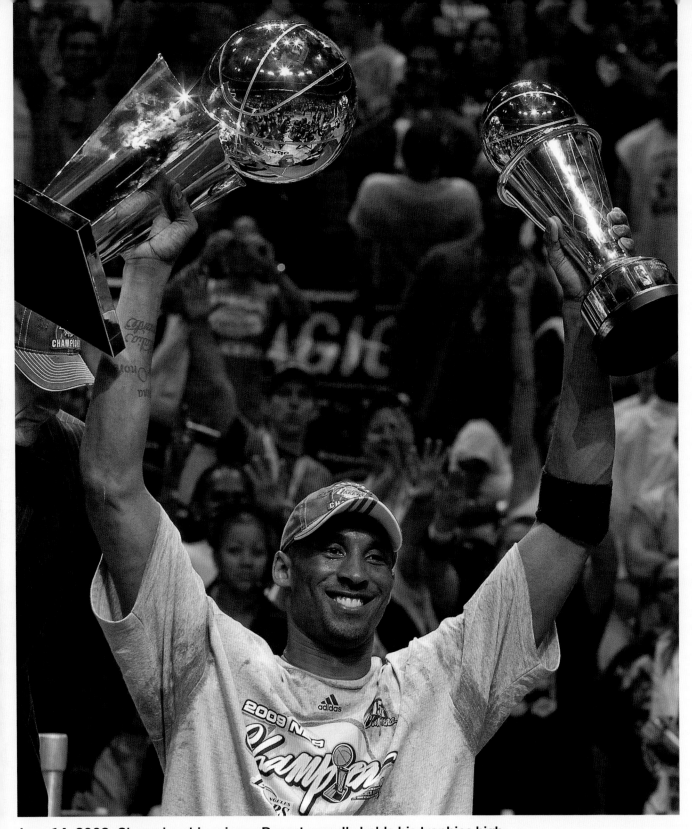

June 14, 2009: Championship-winner Bryant proudly holds his trophies high.

stormed back and clung to a three-point lead with about a minute left. Kobe had the ball when the Celtics double-teamed him. Perhaps in the past, Bryant would have forced the issue himself. Now, though, he found an open teammate, Ron Artest, who nailed an unlikely three-pointer.

Los Angeles won 83–79, giving Bryant his second straight championship and another Finals MVP Award.

Kobe now had five career rings—one more, it should be noted, than Shaquille O'Neal.

MAMBA OUT

The Lakers believed they had what it took to win a third straight championship during the 2010–11 season, and they certainly played like champions for much of the season, going 17–1 during one stretch. Bryant averaged over 25 points per game that season, but his team got swept out of the playoffs in the second round by eventual champions the Dallas Mavericks.

Phil Jackson retired in the offseason, and Los Angeles hired Mike Brown for the 2011–12 season. Bryant would up his scoring average to 27.9 points per game, but the Lakers once again lost in the second round of the playoffs, this time to the Oklahoma City Thunder. The next season, Los Angeles was playing well going into its April 12, 2013, game against the Golden State Warriors. But with just three minutes left, Bryant crumbled to the ground as he drove to the basket, grabbing his left leg. He had torn his Achilles tendon; his season was over.

The 34-year-old Bryant wondered if his entire career was over, writing on Facebook, "Maybe Father Time has defeated me." Instead, he had surgery and attacked his rehab like one would expect from the Black Mamba. He returned to the court in December but almost immediately was hit with another devastating injury—a broken kneecap. As a result, Bryant played in just six games during the 2013–14 season.

The next season, during a December game against the Minnesota Timberwolves, Bryant sank two free throws in the second quarter. The second free throw marked Bryant's 32,293rd career point, and he surpassed Michael Jordan as the third-leading scorer in NBA history.

Unfortunately, that would be the highlight of Bryant's season, as a shoulder injury sustained in January 2015 required surgery.

Now 37 years old, Bryant felt like his body was telling him the end was near. He approached the Players' Tribune—a website founded by former New York Yankees shortstop Derek Jeter—about publishing a poem. This was no ordinary poem, but a love letter to the game of basketball itself. Called "Dear Basketball," the poem also served as Bryant's retirement announcement. The 2015–16 season would be his last. He ended the poem with "Love you always."

And so the 2015–16 season became one long retirement tour, with many teams holding special tributes to Bryant before he played his final game at their respective arenas. The Lakers were one of the worst teams in the league that year, and Kobe was a shell of his former self, averaging just 17 points per game. Still, the legend capped things off in truly spectacular fashion.

Kobe Bryant's last NBA game took place in Los Angeles on April 13, 2016, against the Utah Jazz. After missing his first five shots, Bryant went off, making shot after shot after shot. At the end of the 101–96 Lakers' victory, Bryant had scored an incredible 60 points. Afterward, he addressed the crowd, thanking them for all their support over the years. He then ended his farewell speech with two words: "Mamba out."

April 13, 2016: Bryant plays his last game with the Lakers—a win against the Utah Jazz.

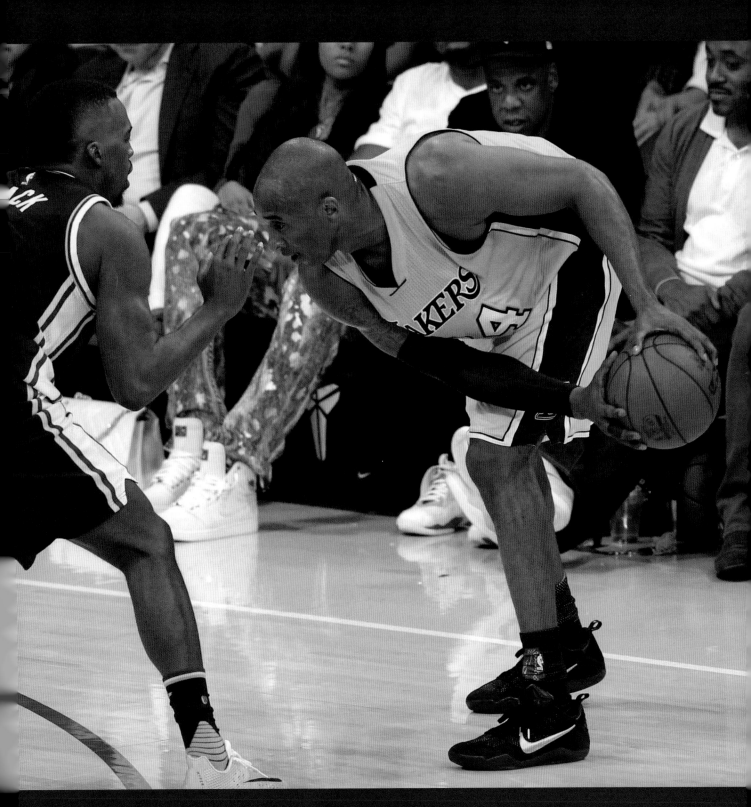

SECOND ACT

To understand the trajectory Kobe's post-NBA life took, you have to go all the way back to his days as a student at Lower Merion High School and, in particular, to his time in Jeanne Mastriano's English class. The witty and charismatic teacher connected with the teenage superstar and through her writing assignments awakened a part of Kobe's personality he didn't know existed.

For one of her assignments, her students had to write a short story for kindergarteners. Kobe, whose mom was constantly on him about his sweaty clothes being strewn all over his bedroom, wrote a story in which those dirty clothes turned into monstrous apparitions that snatched kids from their beds.

Mastriano remained a mentor to Kobe as he moved beyond the walls of Lower Merion and into the bright lights of international fame and success. She no doubt played a role in his decision in 2013 to found a company called Granity Studios, a multimedia company focused on creating novel ways to tell sports-related stories.

One of Granity's projects involved turning Kobe's "Dear Basketball" retirement poem into a short film. Bryant worked with former Disney animator Glen Keane to bring his poem to life. The five-minute film featured drawings by Keane, narration by Bryant, and music by legendary composer John Williams. Released in 2017, the film was critically acclaimed and even received an Academy Award for Best Animated Short Film at the 2018 Oscars. It was the first time a former professional athlete had won an Academy Award.

Later in 2018, Bryant published a book titled *The Mamba Mentality: How I Play*, which consisted of a collection of his thoughts on basketball. The book included an introduction by Phil Jackson and a foreword by Pau Gasol. The next year, Bryant published a novel for kids called *The Wizenard Series: Training Camp*. The book combined basketball with elements of magic. A sequel came out in 2020.

When he wasn't winning Academy Awards or penning bestsellers, Bryant found time to stay connected to the game he loved so much by mentoring the next generation of stars. He helped Boston Celtics All-Star Jayson Tatum develop his mid-range game, and he formed a close relationship with Atlanta Hawks star Trae Young.

Just a few short years into his retirement, and Kobe Bryant had already accomplished more during his second act than most do in their entire careers. "As basketball players we're supposed to shut up and dribble," Bryant once said. "But we do a little more than that."

March 4, 2018: Retired from basketball but not from winning awards, Bryant is presented with an Oscar for his animated short film, *Dear Basketball*.

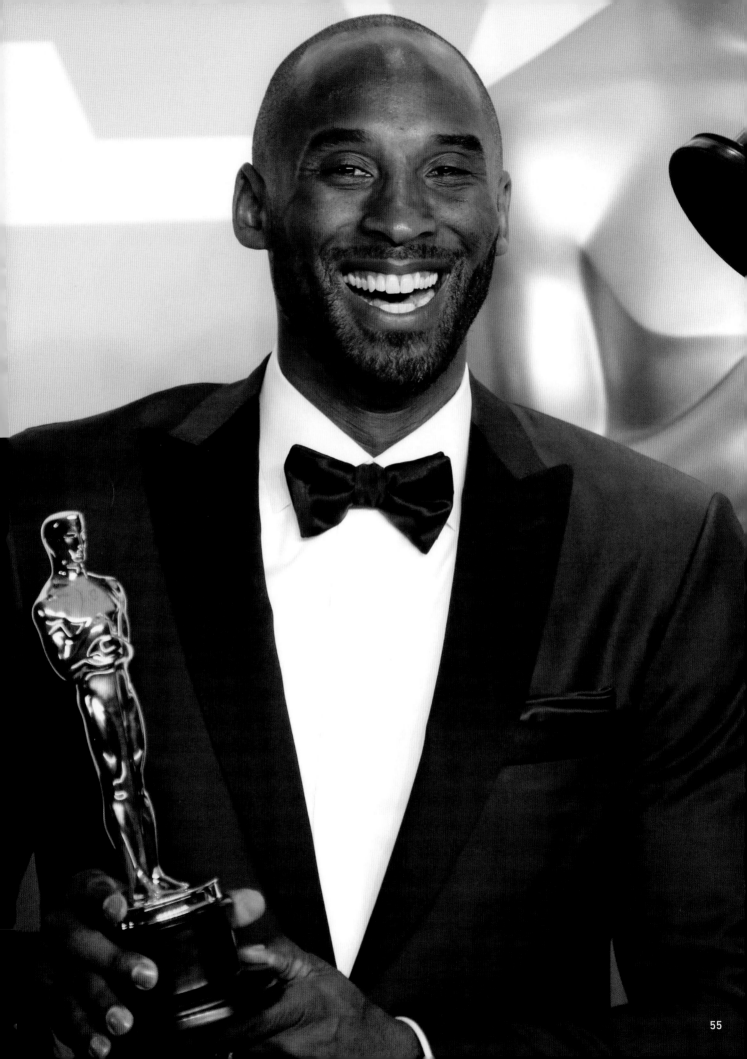

GIRL DAD

Retirement allowed Bryant the opportunity to spend more time with his growing family. When he retired, Kobe and his wife, Vanessa, already had two daughters—Natalia and Gianna. Vanessa gave birth to the couple's third daughter, Bianka, in December 2016. A fourth daughter, Capri, was born in June 2019.

Bryant had met Vanessa Laine back in 1999. At the time, the burgeoning NBA star was considering crossing over into the world of rap. On one occasion, Bryant was filming a rap video when he came across Vanessa, an aspiring model, who was in the same film studio working as a background dancer for a Snoop Dogg video.

Though Bryant's music video and debut rap album were never released, he and Vanessa became a serious couple. In May 2000, after dating for just six months, Kobe asked Vanessa to marry him. She accepted, and the two wed on April 18, 2001, at St. Edward the Confessor Catholic Church in Dana Point, California.

The Bryants' marriage had its share of ups and downs. Things got off to a rocky start because their nuptials caused a rift between Kobe and his parents, who objected to the marriage because Vanessa was just 18 years old at the time (Kobe was 22). When Natalia was born in January 2003, Vanessa urged Kobe to patch things up with his parents, which he did over time.

Bryant's 2003 sexual assault charge brought his relationship with Vanessa to a breaking point. In fact, Vanessa eventually filed for divorce, but the two later reconciled. By the time his playing career came to an

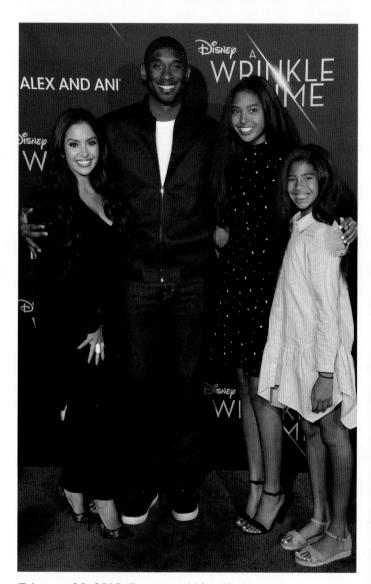

February 26, 2018: Bryant and his wife, Vanessa, and daughters Natalia and Gianna attend the film premiere of *A Wrinkle in Time*.

end, it seemed like those dark times were well in the past, and the Bryants came across as a loving, close-knit family.

Bryant was proud to be a "girl dad," and he often referred to his daughters as his princesses. Though Natalia was a standout volley-

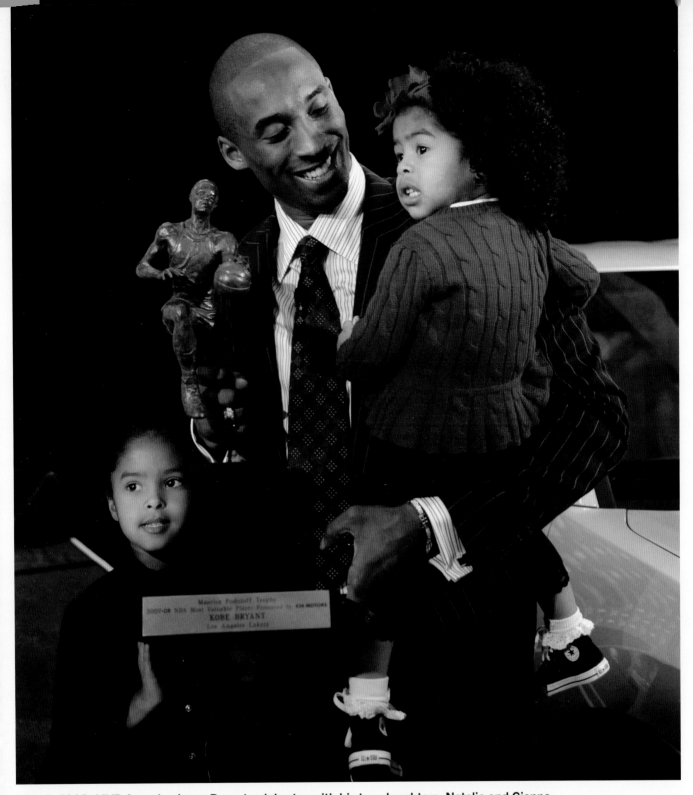

May 6, 2008: MVP Award–winner Bryant celebrates with his two daughters, Natalia and Gianna.

ball player, it was Gianna whose personality was most like her father's. "GiGi" gravitated to basketball at a young age, and she aspired to play the sport professionally.

Bryant opened the Mamba Sports Academy and began coaching his daughter's basketball team. The two were often seen watching games together, GiGi listening intently as Bryant gave

her tips. Sometimes, fans would come up to Kobe and tell him he needed a son to carry on the Bryant family basketball tradition. If they were foolish enough to say this in front of GiGi, the youngster had the confidence to butt in, saying, "No boy for that. I got this."

Tragically, Gianna would never get the opportunity to become a third-generation basketball star.

TRAGEDY AND

On Saturday, January 25, 2020, LeBron James, now a member of the Los Angeles Lakers, passed Bryant on the NBA's all-time scoring list. Bryant congratulated his former rival, posting on Twitter, "Much respect my brother." The next day, Bryant spent the morning at Sunday Mass before heading home to pick up Gianna.

The 13-year-old aspiring basketball star played for her famous father's AAU basketball team, fittingly called Team Mamba. GiGi had a game later that day at a tournament being played at Bryant's Mamba Sports Academy, located 45 miles northwest of Los Angeles.

It was customary for Kobe to travel to his academy by helicopter. On this particular morning, nine people boarded the Sikorsky S-76B helicopter: Bryant, Gianna, six people associated with her team, including two teammates, and the pilot. The aircraft took off from Orange County's John Wayne Airport. Shortly afterward, as the pilot tried to navigate through a layer of thick fog, he lost control, and the helicopter crashed into a hillside. There were no survivors.

News of the 41-year-old's death sent shock-waves across the nation. Back in Philadelphia, Kobe's high school coach Gregg Downer was at home when he first heard the reports of his former star player's death. He prayed the news was wrong before collapsing onto his kitchen floor in despair.

Outside Lower Merion High School, an impromptu shrine sprang up as news of their hero's untimely death spread. The school district put out a statement saying that "Aces Nation has lost its heartbeat." A similar shrine sprouted up outside the Staples Center, the Lak-ers' home arena. NBA teams playing that day honored Kobe by taking either a 24-second shot clock violation or an eight-second backcourt violation. Kobe had worn both No. 24 and No. 8 during his career.

Current and former NBA players displayed shock and sadness. Shaquille O'Neal said there were "no words to express the pain." Once unable to speak to each other, Kobe and Shaq had since patched up their relationship, with Shaq describing Kobe as a little brother.

Kobe and Gianna were laid to rest in a private funeral on February 7. On February 24, a public ceremony was held to commemorate the legend and his daughter, whose dream it was to star in the WNBA. Orange County declared August 24 Kobe Bryant Day. NBA commissioner Adam Silver announced that the All-Star Game MVP Award would from then on be known as the All-Star Game Kobe Bryant MVP Award.

"Kobe was a legend on the court and just getting started in what would have been just as meaningful a second act," former president Barack Obama said. Very few athletes had as big of an impact on the world as Kobe Bean Bryant.

That impact, of course, included his stellar NBA career—5 NBA championships, 18 All-Star appearances, 33,643 career points, 15 All-NBA Team selections, 1 MVP, and induction into the Basketball Hall of Fame. But it also included his off-court contributions as a best-selling author, Academy Award–winning producer, loving father, and setting an overall standard of excellence through his Mamba Mentality.

Because of his everlasting impact, Mamba may be out, but he isn't really gone.

LEGACY

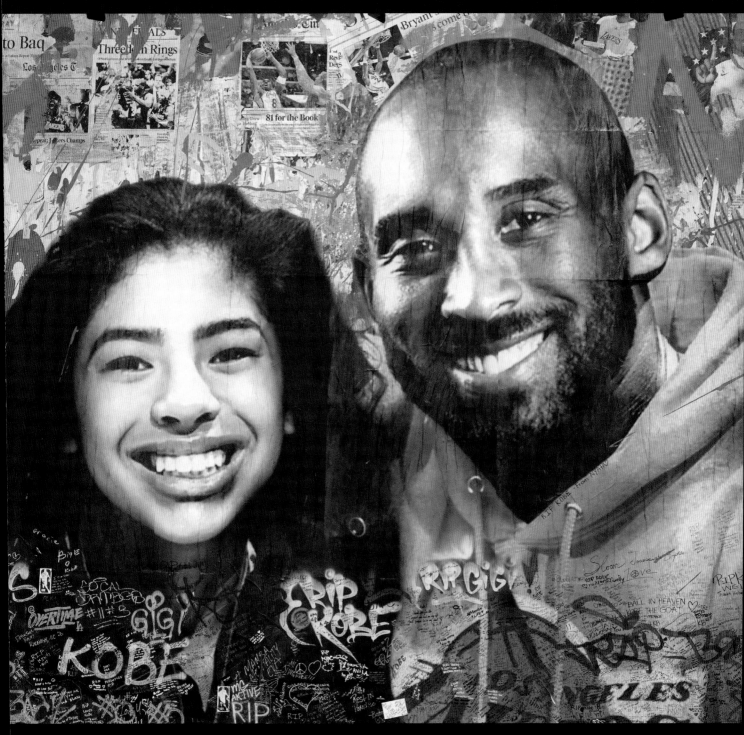

February 16, 2020: A mural in Los Angeles commemorates Kobe and Gianna, who tragically died in a helicopter crash on January 26, 2020.

KOBE BY THE NUMBERS

NBA CHAMPIONSHIPS 5

NBA ALL-STAR APPEARANCES 18

Named a starter each time

ALL-NBA SELECTIONS 15

11 first team, 2 second team, 2 third team

NBA ALL-DEFENSIVE SELECTIONS 12

9 first team,
3 second team

NBA MVP 1

NBA FINALS MVP 2

ALL-STAR MVP 4

OLYMPIC GOLD MEDALS 2

GAMES PLAYED 1,346

15th all-time

MINUTES PLAYED 48,643

8th all-time

CAREER POINTS 33,643

4th all-time

CAREER SCORING AVERAGE 25.0 PPG

16th all-time

NUMBER OF 60-POINT GAMES 6

2nd all-time

CAREER HIGH 8

2nd all-time

STEALS 1,944

16th all-time

GAME-WINNING BUZZER BEATERS 8

Tied 1st with
one franchise

CAREER EARNINGS $328 MILLION

HALL-OF-FAME INDUCTIONS 1

May 15, 2021

May 23, 2012: A confident Kobe smiles during a Lakers game against the Trail Blazers.

DAUGHTERS 4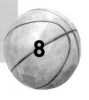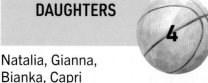

Natalia, Gianna,
Bianka, Capri

ACADEMY AWARDS 1

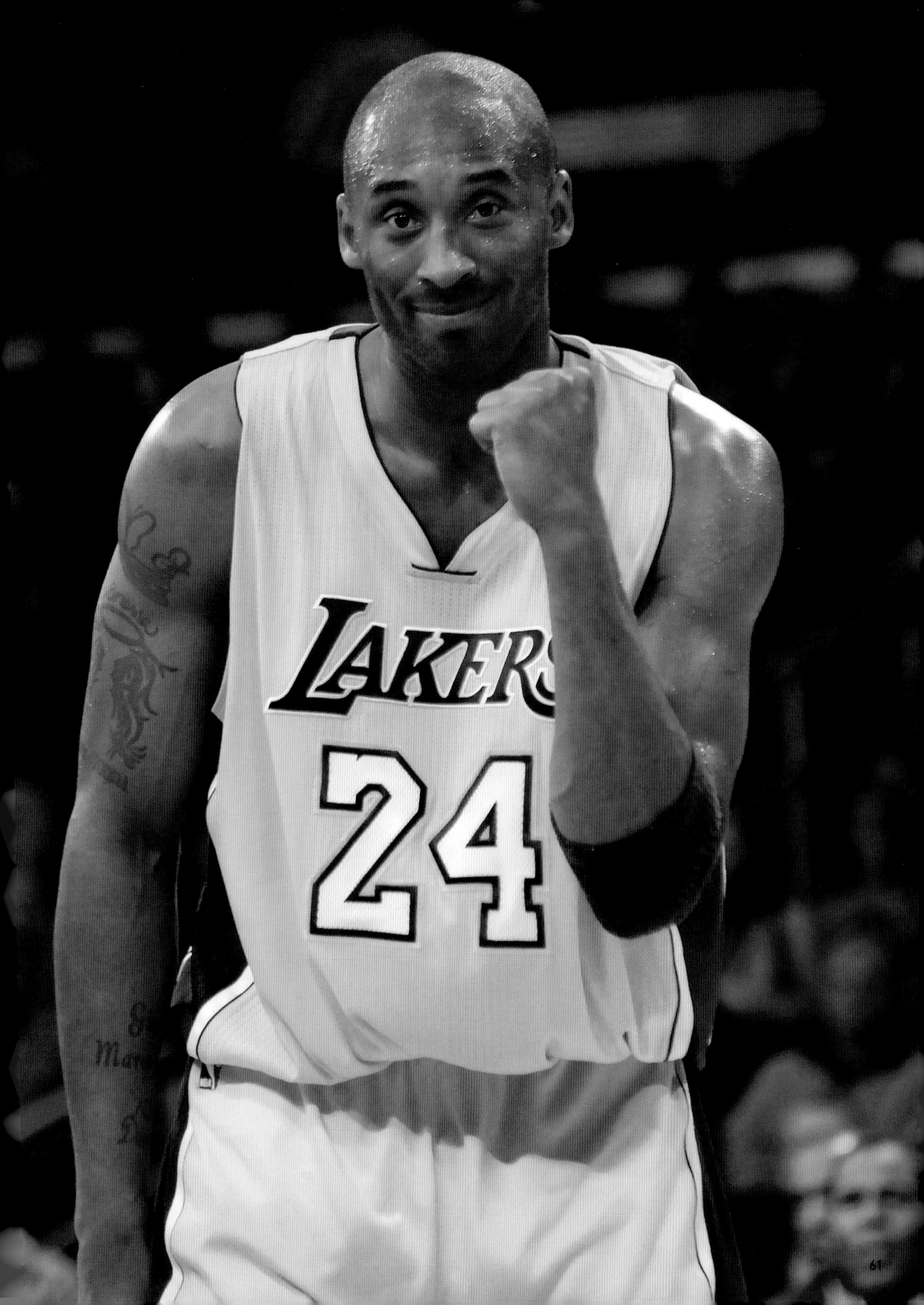
LAKERS
24

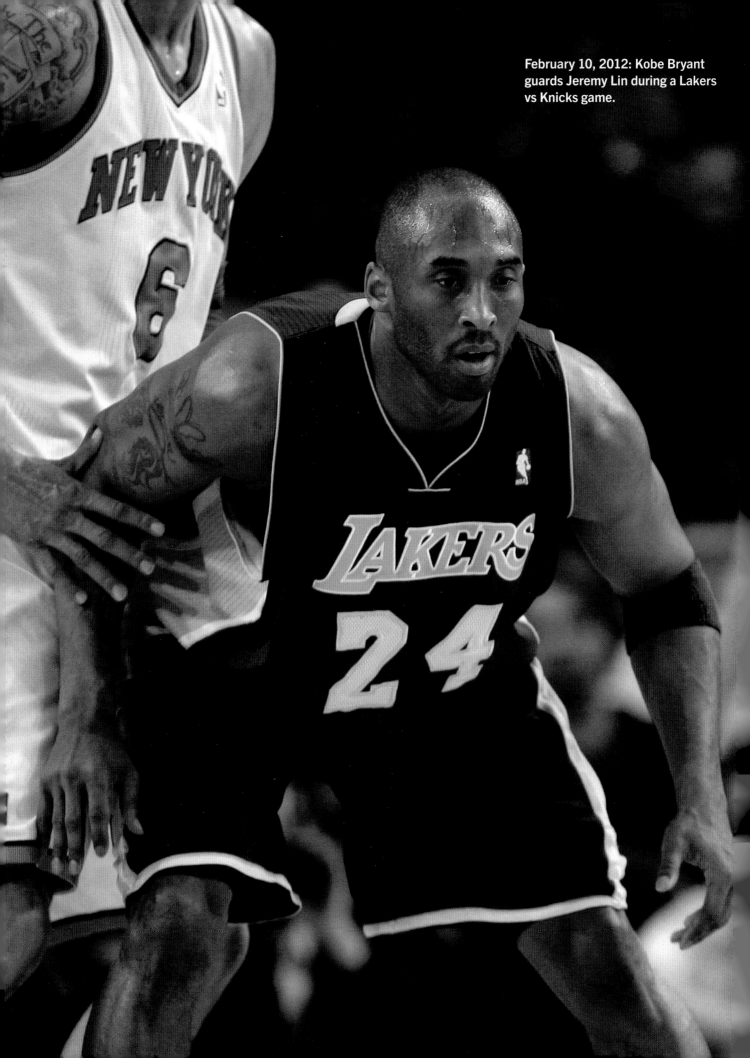

February 10, 2012: Kobe Bryant guards Jeremy Lin during a Lakers vs Knicks game.